ABC OF DIABETES

Fifth Edition

PETER J WATKINS

Honorary Consultant Physician, King's Diabetes Centre, King's College Hospital, London

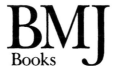
BMJ
Books

© BMJ Publishing Group Ltd 1983, 1988, 1993, 1998, 2003

First edition 1983
Second edition 1988
Third edition 1993
Fourth edition 1998
Fifth edition 2003
Second impression 2004

by BMJ Publishing Group Ltd, BMA House, Tavistock Square,
London WC1H 9JR

www.bmjbooks.com

British Library Cataloguing in Publication Data
A catalogue record for this book is available from the British Library

ISBN 0-7279-16939

Typeset by Newgen Imaging Systems (P) Ltd, Chennai, India.
Printed and bound in Spain by Graphy Cems, Navarra.

The cover image shows molecular graphics of insulin hexamer
with permission of JC Revy/Science Photo Library

Contents

Acknowledgments

Any ideas or inspiration which these pages may contain have inevitably been learnt or borrowed from others. I am indebted to the late Professor JM Malins and Dr MG FitzGerald, through whose enthusiasm I was first introduced to diabetes, and to the late Dr David Pyke through whose energy this interest has been fostered over many years. Close collaboration with colleagues at King's both past and present has made possible many of the joint ventures described here, and I am grateful to them all. Our registrars and research fellows and above all our patients have been a constant source of inspiration.

I am particularly grateful to the many colleagues who have assisted me with the preparation of this book, especially Professor Stephanie Amiel (RD Lawrence Professor of Diabetic Medicine), Dr Michael Edmonds and Dr Stephen Thomas (consultant physicians), Dr Tyrrell Evans (general practitioner), Dr Phin Kon (renal physician), Dr William Marshall (Reader in Clinical Biochemistry), Dr Joanna Raeburn (associate specialist), Ms Helen Reid (Diabetes Specialist Nurse), and Mrs Eileen Turner (Consultant Nurse Specialist).
Dr Simon Page (consultant physician in Nottingham) has helped me considerably by his many valuable comments in reading the manuscript. My wife Mrs Val Watkins has throughout provided me with invaluable support and encouragement.

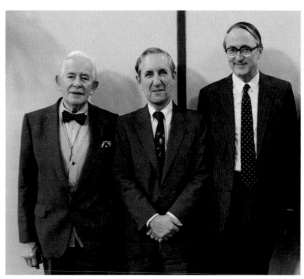

Consultant physicians to the Diabetes Centre at King's from 1938 (from left to right) Dr Wilfred Oakley (1905-1998); Dr David Pyke (1921-2001) and Dr Peter Watkins

Introduction

Advances in clinical science over a single professional lifetime during the second half of the 20th century have led to improvements in understanding the causes and complications of diabetes, together with alleviation of suffering to an extraordinary degree, unimaginable even 25 years ago. Many of the clinical improvements have been initiated at innovative centres across the United Kingdom.

In the 1960s and 1970s physicians had to stand by helplessly watching their patients overwhelmed by complications of the disease. Prevention of blindness by photocoagulation and renal support treatment for those in renal failure became possible in the 1970s, while development of specialist foot clinics during the 1980s succeeded in halving the amputation rate. The sad outcome for pregnancies even 20 years after the discovery of insulin when the fetal mortality rate was more than 25%, has been transformed so that now more than 95% of these pregnancies succeed. And now, the landmark Diabetes Control and Complications Trial (DCCT) of Type 1 diabetes in the United States, and more recently the astonishing achievement of the late Professor Robert Turner in completing the United Kingdom Perspective Diabetes Survey (UKPDS) of Type 2 diabetes have demonstrated how to reduce the incidence and progression of diabetic complications by good treatment.

Yet there is still more. The present technology of managing diabetes was undreamt of until the last quarter of the 20th century. The introduction of home blood glucose monitoring with new non-invasive technologies now in sight, has made possible the achievement of "tight control", while at the same time advances in understanding and reversing diminished awareness of hypoglycaemia are reducing its hazards. The invention of insulin pens and more recently the development of insulin pumps has contributed in great measure to improving the quality of life of those with the burden of lifelong diabetes. Furthermore after the British discoveries of the chemical (Frederick Sanger, 1955) and physical structure (Dorothy Hodgkin, 1969) of insulin followed by the revolution in molecular science, man-made insulin analogues have been introduced, giving further advantages in achieving good blood glucose control while minimising hypoglycaemia.

The initially controversial "invention" of the diabetes specialist nurse by Dr Joan Walker in Leicester in the 1950s is arguably one of the most important advances in health care, not only for those with diabetes but across the whole of medicine. The tremendous benefits in the delivery of care especially to those with diabetes and other chronic diseases have been accompanied by recognition of community needs and improvements in crossing the primary/secondary care interface. It is now to be hoped that improvements in information technology, more sophisticated audit, and provision of a national eye screening programme may emerge from the National Service Framework of 2002/2003.

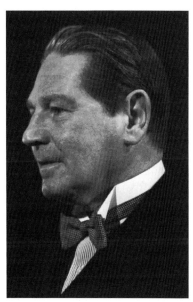

RD Lawrence 1892-1968. Founder of the diabetic clinic at King's in the 1920s, founder of the British Diabetic Association in 1934

Rapid clinical advances of this magnitude require substantial support. Diabetes UK, founded as the Diabetic Association by Dr RD Lawrence and his patient HG Wells in 1934 (later the British Diabetic Association), has uniquely supported both patients and their needs as well as clinical and scientific research. More recently the Juvenile Diabetes Foundation has made substantial contributions. Furthermore the pharmaceutical industry has been both innovative in its own laboratories as well as supportive of both patients and clinicians.

It gives particular pleasure to reproduce some parts of the personal account by Mrs B-J (with her permission) of her own diabetes over the last 70 years of attendances at King's College Hospital. She describes vividly aspects of treatment and some of the problems faced by people with diabetes, and one can see clearly how many improvements there have been during her lifetime. Her account should give tremendous encouragement to those now starting on their own life with diabetes.

The ABC is intended as a strictly practical guide to the management of diabetes and its complications and is directed to all those doctors, nurses, and health professionals, other than established specialists, who see diabetic patients, and medical students should find some value in its pages. Many of the innovations of the end of the 20th century are described in this fifth edition of the ABC in the hope that it will help in the delivery of the very best standards of care to those who need it in the 21st century.

1 What is diabetes?

Diabetes once diagnosed is for life. The perseverance and self discipline needed over a lifetime can often tax even the most robust of people to the limit. Those caring for them also require perseverance and an understanding of humanity combined with a cautious optimism, to guide those with diabetes through the peaks and troughs of their lives.

Definition

Diabetes occurs either because of a lack of insulin or because of the presence of factors that oppose the action of insulin. The result of insufficient action of insulin is an increase in blood glucose concentration (hyperglycaemia). Many other metabolic abnormalities occur, notably an increase in ketone bodies in the blood when there is a severe lack of insulin.

Diagnosis

The diagnosis of diabetes must always be established by a blood glucose measurement made in an accredited laboratory.

Glucose tolerance test

The glucose tolerance test is not normally needed in routine clinical practice, and then only if uncertainty exists in younger patients, or to establish an exact diagnosis in pregnancy. For reliable results, glucose tolerance tests should be performed in the morning after an overnight fast, with the patient sitting quietly and not smoking; it is also important that the patient should have normal meals for the previous three days and should not have been dieting. False results may also occur if the patient has been ill recently or has had prolonged bed rest. Blood glucose concentrations are measured fasting and then one and two hours after a drink of 75 g of glucose in 250-350 ml water (in children 1·75 g/kg to a maximum of 75 g), preferably flavoured, for example, with pure lemon juice. Urine tests should be performed before the glucose drink and at one and two hours. Interpretation of blood glucose values according to WHO criteria is shown in the table.

Gestational diabetes
This term embraces the criteria for both diabetes and impaired glucose tolerance when discovered during pregnancy (see page 80).
   Glucose tolerance tests may also show:
   Renal glycosuria—this occurs when there is glycosuria but normal blood glucose concentrations; this is a benign condition, only rarely indicating unusual forms of renal disease. It is worth issuing these patients with a certificate to prevent them from being subjected to repeated glucose tolerance tests at every medical examination.
   Steeple or lag curve—this is described when fasting and two hour concentrations are normal, but those between are high, causing glycosuria; this is also a benign condition, which most commonly occurs after gastrectomy but may occur in healthy people.

Impaired glucose tolerance
This is defined in the table. Patients are managed at the discretion of the physician. In general, no treatment is given to

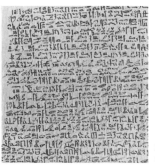

Ebers papyrus: early clinical description of diabetes (Egyptian, 1500 BC)

WHO criteria for the diagnosis of diabetes

1 Symptoms of diabetes plus casual venous *plasma* glucose ≥ 11·1 mmol/l. Casual is defined as any time of day without regard to time since last meal. The classic symptoms of diabetes include polyuria, polydipsia, and unexplained weight loss
2 Fasting *plasma* glucose ≥ 7·0 mmol/l or whole blood ≥ 6·1 mmol/l. Fasting is defined as no calorie intake for at least 8 hours
3 2 hour *plasma* glucose ≥ 11·1 mmol/l during oral glucose tolerance test using 75 g glucose load

In the absence of symptoms, these criteria should be confirmed by repeat testing on a different day. If the fasting or random values are not diagnostic, the 2 hour value post-glucose load should be used

Note.
Fasting plasma glucose < 6·1 mmol/l—normal
Fasting plasma glucose ≥ 6·1 and < 7·0 mmol/l—impaired fasting blood glucose
Fasting plasma glucose ≥ 7·0 mmol/l—provisional diagnosis of diabetes; the diagnosis must be confirmed (see above)

Adapted from *Diabetes Care* 1997;20:1183-1195

Glucose tolerance test

	Glucose concentration (mmol/l)		
	Venous whole blood	Capillary whole blood	Venous plasma
*Diabetes mellitus**			
Fasting	≥ 6·1	≥ 6·1	≥ 7·0
2 hours after glucose load	≥ 10·0	≥ 11·1	≥ 11·1
Impaired glucose tolerance			
Fasting	< 6·1	< 6·1	< 7·0
2 hours after glucose load	≥ 6·7 < 10·0	≥ 7·8 < 11·1	≥ 7·8 < 11·1

*In the absence of symptoms at least one additional abnormal blood glucose concentration is needed to confirm clinical diagnosis—for example, 1 hour value of 11 mmol/l or more

elderly people, but diet, exercise and weight reduction are advisable in younger subjects. Over 10 years, approximately half of those with impaired glucose tolerance will develop diabetes, one-quarter will persist with impaired glucose tolerance, and one-quarter will revert to normal. Pregnant women with "impaired glucose tolerance" must be treated as if they were diabetic; for interpretation of the test in pregnancy seen page 80.

Types of diabetes

Type 1 diabetes (previously insulin dependent diabetes) is due to B-cell destruction, usually leading to absolute insulin deficiency). It can be immune mediated or idiopathic.

Type 2 diabetes (previously non-insulin dependent diabetes) ranges from those with predominant insulin resistance associated with relative insulin deficiency, to those with a predominantly insulin secretory defect with insulin resistance.

Type 1 and Type 2 diabetes are the commonest forms of primary diabetes mellitus. The division is important both clinically in assessing the need for treatment, and also in understanding the causes of diabetes which are entirely different in the two groups.

Type 1 diabetes

Type 1 diabetes is due to destruction of B-cells in the pancreatic islets of Langerhans with resulting loss of insulin production. A combination of environmental and genetic factors that trigger an autoimmune attack on the B-cells is responsible, occurring in genetically susceptible individuals. Thus, among monozygotic identical twins only about one-third of the pairs are concordant for diabetes in contrast to the situation in Type 2 diabetes where almost all pairs are concordant. The process of islet destruction probably begins very early in life and is known to start several years before the clinical onset of diabetes.

HLA status

The major histocompatibility complex antigens are adjuncts to several types of immunological activity. Ninety percent of Type 1 diabetic patients show either DR3 or DR4, or both together, while DR2 is protective against diabetes.

Autoantibodies and cellular immunity

Islet cell antibodies are present at diagnosis in most Type 1 diabetic patients and gradually decline and disappear during the following years. Antibodies to specific proteins have more recently been identified: these include antibodies to glutamic acid decarboxylase (GAD, a 64-kDa antigen); and even closer association is found in the presence of antibodies to tyrosine phosphatase (37 kDa, IA-2). The presence in a non-diabetic individual of three or more antibodies (islet cell antibodies, anti-GAD antibodies, anti-IA-2 antibodies, anti-insulin autoantibodies) indicates an 88% chance of developing diabetes within 10 years.

The presence of insulinitis at the onset of Type 1 diabetes represents the role of inflammatory cells (for example, cytotoxic T cells and macrophages) in B-cell destruction. Macrophages also produce cytokines leading to activation of lymphocytes known to be present at the onset of Type 1 diabetes.

Attempts have been made to prevent the onset of Type 1 diabetes. Immune suppression can to some extent preserve islet function, but permanent remissions are not normally achieved and the treatment is in any case too dangerous for routine use.

Other specific types of diabetes

- *Genetic defects of β cell function*—chromosome 12 hepatic nuclear factor-1α (HNF-1α) (formerly maturity onset diabetes of the young (MODY) 3), chromosome 7 glucokinase defect (formerly MODY 2), chromosome 20 HNF-4α (formerly MODY 1), mitochondrial DNA mutation
- *Genetic defects in insulin action*—Type A insulin resistance (genetic defects in insulin receptor), lipoatrophic diabetes, genetic defects in the PPARγ receptor
- *Gestational diabetes*
- *Diseases of the exocrine pancreas*—pancreatitis, pancreatectomy, carcinoma of pancreas, cystic fibrosis, fibro-calculous pancreatopathy, haemochromatosis
- *Endocrinopathies*—acromegaly, Cushing's disease, Conn's syndrome, glucagonoma, phaeochromocytoma, somatostatinoma
- *Drug induced* (these agents in particular exacerbate hyperglycaemia in patients with established diabetes)—corticosteroids, diazoxide, β adrenergic agonists (for example, intravenous salbutamol), thiazides, α interferon
- *Uncommon forms of immune mediated diabetes*—stiff man syndrome, anti-insulin receptor antibodies (Type B insulin resistance)
- *Infections*—congenital rubella, cytomegalovirus
- *Other genetic syndromes sometimes associated with diabetes*—Wolfram syndrome, Down's syndrome, Turner's syndrome, Klinefelter's syndrome, Prader-Willi syndrome

Comparison of Type 1 and Type 2 diabetes

Type 1 diabetes	Type 2 diabetes
Inflammatory reaction in islets	No insulitis
Islet B-cells destroyed	B-cells function
Islet cell antibodies	No islet cell antibodies
HLA related	Not HLA related
Not directly inherited	Strong genetic basis (some cases)

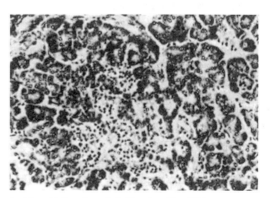

An islet with lymphocytic infiltration (insulitis)

The use of nicotinamide to prevent diabetes by altering macrophage function has not proved to be of benefit. Giving insulin itself may conserve islet function; the results of trials are awaited.

Associated autoimmune disorders
The incidence of coeliac disease, Addison's disease, hypothyroidism, and pernicious anaemia are increased in Type 1 diabetic patients, and appear to occur especially in those with persisting islet cell antibodies.

Risks of inheriting diabetes
A child of a mother with Type 1 diabetes has an increased risk of developing the same type of diabetes, amounting to 1-2% by 25 years; the risk is about three times greater if the father has this disease. If both parents have the disease the risk is further increased and genetic counselling should be sought by these rare couples.

Type 2 diabetes
There are numerous causes of Type 2 diabetes, which is now known to include a wide range of disorders with differing progression and outlook. The underlying mechanism is due either to diminished insulin secretion—that is, an islet defect, associated with increased peripheral resistance to the action of insulin resulting in decreased peripheral glucose uptake, or increased hepatic glucose output. Probably as many as 98% of Type 2 diabetic patients are "idiopathic"—that is, no specific causative defect has been identified. Whether decreasing insulin secretion or increasing insulin resistance occurs first is still uncertain, but the sequence of events may vary in different individuals. Obesity is the commonest cause of insulin resistance. Other rare insulin resistant states are shown in the table.

Some adults (especially those not overweight) over 25 years of age who appear to present with Type 2 diabetes may have latent autoimmune diabetes of adulthood (LADA) and become insulin dependent. Autoantibodies are often present in this group of patients.

Type 2 diabetes is a slowly progressive disease: insulin secretion declines over several decades, resulting in an insidious deterioration of glycaemic control which becomes increasingly difficult to achieve.

Obesity
Relative insulin resistance occurs in obese subjects, perhaps because of down regulation of insulin receptors due to hyperinsulinaemia. Obese subjects have a considerably increased risk of developing Type 2 diabetes. Fat distribution is relevant to the development of diabetes, so that those who are "apple shaped" (android obesity, waist-hip ratio > 0.9) are more prone to Type 2 diabetes than those who are "pear shaped" (gynoid obesity, waist-hip ratio < 0.7).

The importance of leptin in the evolution of lifestyle related obesity is unclear. Leptin is a single chain peptide produced by adipose tissue and its receptors are expressed widely throughout the brain and peripheral tissues; when injected into leptin deficient rodents it causes profound hypophagia and weight loss. Plasma leptin levels rise in parallel with body fat content. Although very rare cases of morbid obesity due to leptin deficiency have been reported, and are shown to respond to leptin injections, there is in general an absence of measurable biological responses to leptin, which at present has no role in the management of obesity.

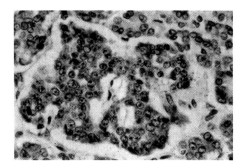

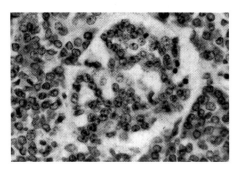

A pancreatic islet after 50 years of Type 1 diabetes: (Top) in this slide A-cells stained for glucagon are intact; (Bottom) in this slide, which is stained for insulin, B-cells are completely absent

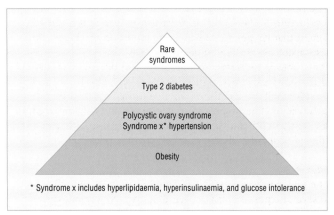

Insulin resistance and disease

Increased risk for Type 2 diabetes
- People over 40 years of age
- People of Asian or African-Caribbean ethnic origin
- Overweight people
- Family history of diabetes
- History of gestational diabetes
- History of large baby (birth weight exceeding 4 kg)

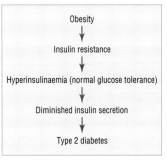

Natural history of Type 2 diabetes

ABC of Diabetes

Birthweight and Type 2 diabetes
Recent observations suggest a relationship between low birthweight and the development in middle age of insulin resistance, Type 2 diabetes, and coronary artery disease. Those who are smallest at birth and largest at one year of age are most at risk.

Genetics of Type 2 diabetes
Type 2 diabetes has a strong genetic component, manifest in the high concordance of diabetes in monozygotic twins, familial clustering and differences in prevalence between ethnic groups. An increasing number of specific genetic defects are becoming recognised and some are described below.

Type 2 diabetes in children and young people
Hitherto, childhood diabetes was witnessed in some ethnic minorities and in those with the rare inherited MODY syndromes described below. Growing recognition now exists of a substantial increase of this disease in the prosperous industrialised nations. In the United States, between 8% and 45% of recently diagnosed cases of diabetes among children and adolescents are Type 2, and the problem is increasing. It is most likely to occur at 12 to 14 years of age, more frequently in girls, and is strongly associated with obesity, physical inactivity and a family history of Type 2 diabetes. When young people of lean physique are discovered to have Type 2 diabetes, it is important to attempt to identify whether they may represent those with LADA and thus in need of insulin. There is also evidence that in approximately one-quarter of such patients diabetes is due to a specific genetic defect including those of the MODY group described below or other rare genetic syndromes.

Dominantly inherited Type 2 diabetes (MODY)
Seven genetic syndromes, three of which are shown in the box at the top of page 2, cause MODY—defined as an early onset of dominantly inherited Type 2 diabetes. Two (or at the very least one) members of such families should have been diagnosed before 25 years of age, three generations (usually first-degree) should have diabetes, and they should not normally require insulin until they have had diabetes for more than five years.

Mitochondrial diabetes
Mitochondrial diabetes and deafness is a rare form of diabetes maternally transmitted, and is related to the A3243G mitochondrial DNA mutation. Diabetes is diagnosed in the fourth to fifth decades, usually in thin patients with symptoms. Patients respond better to sulphonylureas than to diet alone. Diabetic microvascular complications do occur.

Insulin resistant diabetes
Some rare insulin resistant states exist in which hundreds or even thousands of units of insulin may be ineffective. They are often associated with lipodystrophy, hyperlipidaemia, and acanthosis nigricans. Type A insulin resistance is due to genetic defects in the insulin receptor or in the post-receptor pathway. Type B insulin resistance occurs as a result of IgG autoantibodies directed against the insulin receptor; it is often associated with other autoimmune disorders such as systemic lupus erythematosis, and it is much commoner in women of African descent. Management of these conditions can be very difficult and specialist texts should be consulted.

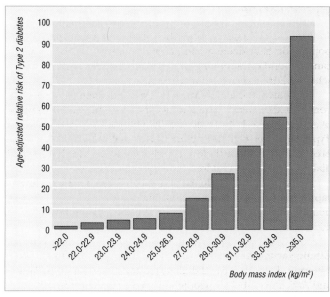

Relative risk of Type 2 diabetes according to body mass index in US women aged 30 to 55 years

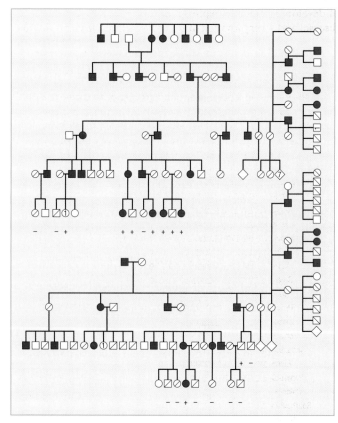

A family with dominantly inherited Type 2 diabetes. HNF-1α defect (chromosome 12), formerly MODY 3. Diabetic patients are shown in black

Prevalence

In the United Kingdom more than three percent of the population have diabetes, and about the same number again can be found on screening in population studies. Among schoolchildren about two in 1000 have diabetes.

Diabetes can occur at any age. Type 2 diabetes is most common after middle age and occurs most often at 50-70 years of age, affecting both sexes equally. The peak incidence of Type 1 diabetes is at 10-12 years with a small male predominance. Nevertheless, elderly people can also have Type 1 diabetes, and some children have Type 2 diabetes.

Worldwide, the incidence of Type 2 diabetes is increasing rapidly: in 1995, it was estimated that there were 135 million people with diabetes, this may rise to about 300 million by 2025, increasing particularly in developing countries.

Ethnic variations

The prevalence of Type 2 diabetes is particularly high in Asian and African-Caribbean people and presents a considerable health burden in some inner urban areas. Thus in the United Kingdom 20% of Asians and 17% of African-Caribbeans over 40 years of age have Type 2 diabetes. Children not infrequently have Type 2 diabetes. Asian people have a particularly high risk of developing diabetic nephropathy and coronary artery disease, and a very low risk of foot ulceration; those among the

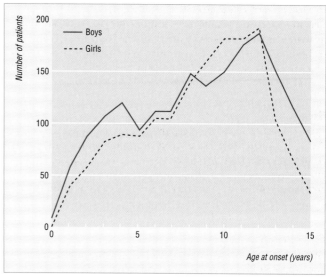

Age of onset of Type 1 diabetes in 3537 children from the British Diabetic Association (now Diabetes UK) register

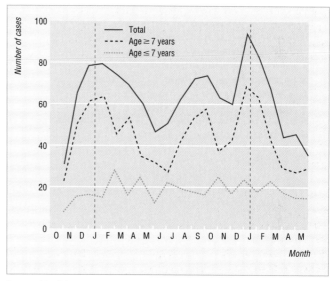

Seasonal incidence of the onset of Type 1 diabetes showing that nearly three times as many of the older children develop the disorder in the winter months, suggesting some role for viral infections

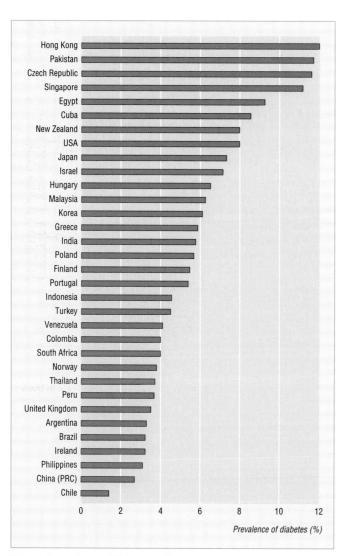

Estimated prevalence of diabetes mellitus in selected countries in 2000

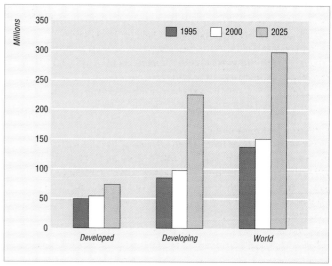

Number of people aged ≥ 20 years estimated to have Type 2 diabetes in developed and developing countries

5

black races are prone to severe hypertension that can be difficult to treat, and also have a strong tendency to develop gestational diabetes.

Prevention of Type 2 diabetes

Lifestyle changes in those prone to Type 2 diabetes can effectively delay the onset of this disease. Several studies in different countries have demonstrated the feasibility of achieving this by a programme of weight reduction, improved diet (less fat, less saturated fat, and more dietary fibre) and increased physical activity. Recent investigations show that the development of diabetes can be approximately halved if these lifestyle changes are maintained over four years.

Diabetic complications

Patients with long-standing diabetes, both Type 1 and Type 2, may develop complications affecting the eyes, kidneys or nerves (microvascular complications) or major arteries. The major arteries are affected in people with diabetes, causing a substantial increase both in coronary artery disease and strokes as well as peripheral vascular disease. The greatest risk of large vessel disease occurs in those diabetic patients who develop proteinuria or microalbuminuria, which is associated with widespread vascular damage. The distribution of arterial narrowing tends to be more distal than in non-diabetic people, whether in coronary arteries or in the peripheral arteries affecting feet and legs. Medial arterial calcification (Monckeberg's sclerosis) is also substantially increased in patients with neuropathy and in those with renal impairment. The functional effects of vascular calcification are uncertain.

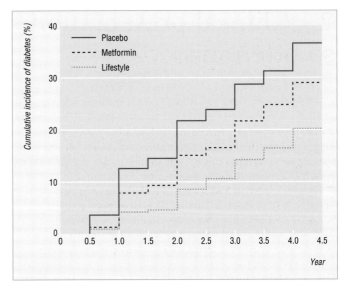

Cumulative incidence of diabetes according to the Diabetes Prevention Programme Research Group. The diagnosis of diabetes was based on the criteria of the American Diabetes Association. The incidence of diabetes differed significantly among the three groups (P < 0.001 for each comparison), showing that lifestyle interventions are particularly effective in diminishing the development of Type 2 diabetes

2 Clinical presentation: why is diabetes so often missed?

Thirst, tiredness, pruritus vulvae or balanitis, polyuria, and weight loss are the familiar symptoms of diabetes. Why then is the diagnosis so often missed? Of 15 new patients with diabetes presenting in our diabetic ward for the first time with ketoacidosis, 14 had had no tests for diabetes after a total of 41 visits to their doctors. Almost all these serious cases of ketoacidosis could have been prevented.

Patients do not, of course, always describe their symptoms in the clearest possible terms, or else their complaints may occur only as an indirect consequence of the more common features. Many patients describe dry mouth rather than thirst, and patients have been investigated for dysphagia when dehydration was the cause. Polyuria is often treated blindly with antibiotics; it may cause enuresis in young people and incontinence in elderly people and the true diagnosis is often overlooked. Complex urological investigations and even circumcision are sometimes performed before diabetes is considered.

Confusion in diagnosis

Some diabetic patients present chiefly with weight loss, but even then the diagnosis is sometimes missed, and I have seen two teenagers referred for psychiatric management of anorexia nervosa before admission with ketoacidosis. Perhaps weakness, tiredness, and lethargy, which may be the dominant symptoms, are the most commonly misinterpreted; "tonics" and iron are sometimes given as the symptoms worsen.

Deteriorating vision is not uncommon as a presentation, due either to change of refraction causing myopia (mainly in Type 1 diabetes) or to the early development of retinopathy (mainly in Type 2 diabetes). Foot ulceration or sepsis in older patients brings them to accident and emergency departments and is nearly always due to diabetes. Occasionally painful neuropathy is the presenting symptom, causing extreme pain in the feet, thighs, or trunk.

Glycosuria itself is responsible for the monilial overgrowth which causes pruritus vulvae or balanitis; some older men are first aware of diabetes when they notice white spots on their trousers. In hot climates drops of sugary urine attract an interested population of ants, and at least one patient now attending the clinic at King's College Hospital presented in this way before he came to England.

Patterns of presentation

Symptoms are similar in the two types of diabetes (Type 1 and Type 2), but they vary in their intensity. The presentation is most typical and the symptoms develop most rapidly in patients with Type 1 diabetes; they usually develop over some weeks, but the duration may be a few days to a few months. There is usually considerable weight loss and exhaustion. If the diagnosis is missed, diabetic ketoacidosis occurs. Type 1 diabetes occurs under 40 years of age in approximately 70% of cases but can occur at any age, and even in older people.

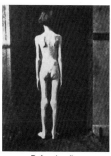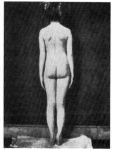
Before insulin   Four months after insulin

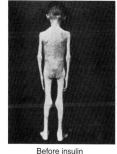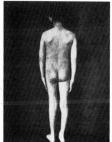
Before insulin   After insulin

Insulin dependent diabetes, 1922

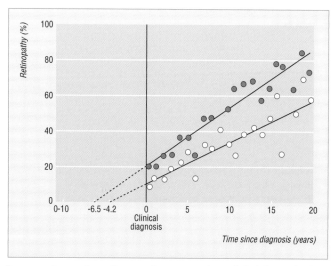

Presence of any retinopathy according to years since clinical diagnosis of Type 2 diabetes among patients in Southern Wisconsin (●) and rural Western Australia (○). Solid lines represent data fitted by weighted regression; lines are extrapolated to indicate the time at which onset of observable retinopathy is estimated to have occurred, demonstrating that diabetes was likely to have been present for several years before the clinical diagnosis was made

Presenting symptoms (%) in 547 consecutive cases of diabetes seen by Professor John Malins

				Symptoms							
Age	Males	Females	Total	None	Thirst	Wasting	Fatigue	Pruritus vulvae	Sepsis	Visual	Other
0-39	28	27	55	9	62	14	4	9	2		
40-59	98	108	206	22	22	9	9	21(2)*	7	6	4
60+	100	186	286	22	22	5	8	22(6)*	6	10	5

*Cases of balanitis in males

Symptoms in patients with Type 2 diabetes are similar but tend to be insidious in their onset; sometimes these patients deny any symptoms, although they often admit to feeling more energetic after treatment has been started. These patients are usually middle aged or elderly, but increasingly children, especially those of ethnic minorities, or those who are inert and overweight, are developing Type 2 diabetes. Microvascular and macrovascular complications are frequently already present when Type 2 diabetes is diagnosed. Type 2 diabetes is commonly detected at routine medical examinations or on admission to hospital with another illness.

> **Type 2 diabetes—presentations**
> * Diabetic symptoms   53%
> * Incidental   29%
> * Infections   16%
>   (for example, candida)
> * Diabetic complications   2%

Identifying patients in need of insulin

Patients in need of treatment with insulin must be identified early. This is done by judging the patient's clinical features; blood glucose concentrations alone offer a relatively poor guide, although most patients with a blood glucose concentration greater than 25 mmol/l are likely to need insulin.

Features suggesting need for insulin are:

* a rapid development of symptoms
* substantial weight loss—patients are usually thin and demonstrate a dry tongue or more severe dehydration
* weakness
* the presence of ketonuria.

If their condition worsens, vomiting can occur and they rapidly become ketoacidotic; these patients are drowsy, dehydrated, overbreathing, and their breath smells of acetone (although many people are unable to detect this smell).

The following groups of patients are likely to need insulin:

* almost all children and most of those under 30-40 years of age
* women who present during pregnancy
* diabetic patients whose tablet treatment has failed
* all patients who have undergone pancreatectomy.

If there is any doubt give insulin. It can never be wrong to do so, and if the decision was mistaken it can easily be reversed.

> **Identifying patients in need of insulin**
>
> *Symptoms*
> * Rapid onset
> * Substantial weight loss
> * Weakness
> * Vomiting
>
> *Signs*
> * Usually thin
> * Dry tongue
> * Weak
>
> *Ketoacidosis*
> * Drowsiness
> * Dehydration
> * Overbreathing
> * Breath smelling of acetone
>
> *Age*
> * Any, more likely under 30 years
>
> *Blood glucose concentration*
> * Any
>
> *Other indications*
> * When tablets have failed during pregnancy
> * When diet has failed during intercurrent illness
> * In patients who have undergone pancreatomy
>
> * Ill patients need admission
> * Others may start insulin at home
> * If there is any doubt use insulin

Opportunistic screening

The diagnosis of diabetes should no longer be missed. New patients attending their doctor, whether the family doctor, at a hospital outpatient clinic or accident and emergency department, should have a blood glucose measurement as a matter of routine, especially if their symptoms are unexplained. Only a few diabetic patients are wholly without symptoms and their diabetes should be detected by screening at any medical examination. Opportunistic screening for diabetes in this way is a duty.

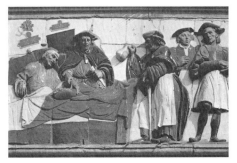

Della Robbia panel from the Ospedale del Ceppo, Pistoia, 1514

The personal story of Mrs B-J's diabetes

Mrs B-J was born in 1922 and developed Type 1 diabetes at the age of 10 years in 1932. She saw Dr RD Lawrence at diagnosis and in 1989 wrote an account of her own diabetes which will be presented over several chapters in this book.

Presentation and diagnosis

I was always a lively, energetic child so nobody was particularly surprised when I seemed to be growing tall and thin at the end of the summer of 1932. Because of my weight loss, my mother took me to our family doctor who thought I might have TB. He told her to put me to bed for one week, then take me back to him with a urine specimen. Up till then I was perfectly fit and well, but being in bed without exercise, I soon lost my appetite and only wanted oranges and drinks. At night, my mother put water in several quart milk bottles by my bed, but I had drunk it all— about ten pints—before my parents came up to bed. This meant dozens of trips to the toilet each night as a chamber pot could not cope with it.

After about three days, my mother went back to the doctor with a specimen and he said that I had diabetes and must go into hospital the next day. My mother was upset but also relieved, as she had a deep fear of TB.

That night a neighbour called to see how I was. My mother did not realise that I could hear their conversation and told her what was wrong. In a loud, shocked voice this lady asked, "Is she going to die?" I was immediately interested, and hearing my mother say that I wouldn't if I did not eat sweets, cake, biscuits, etc. for the rest of my life, I resolved there and then that I would do just that. I never wanted again to feel as awful as I did just then. I think that eavesdropping probably affected me for the rest of my life, and since then I have had no desire for sweet things except as part of my diet, or for warding off hypos.

The next morning my parents took me by taxi to King's College Hospital.

The first illustration is from Geyelin, HR, Marrop, C. *J Med Res* 1922;2:767-9. The figure showing presence of retinopathy according to years since diagnosis is adapted from *Diab Care* 1992;15:815-21 with permission of American Diabetes Association. The table showing presenting symptoms of diabetes is adapted from Malins J. *Clinical diabetes mellitus.* London: Eyre and Spottiswoode, 1968, and the box showing Type 2 diabetes presentation uses data from UKPDS. *Diabetes Med* 1998;5:154-9.

3 Aims of treatment: a healthy lifestyle

Diabetes is easy to diagnose, but can be managed with negligent ease by those inclined to do so RB Tattersall, 1990

The first concerns in treating diabetic patients are to save life, alleviate symptoms, and enhance the quality of an independent life. Thereafter treatment aims to minimise the long-term complications and reduce early mortality.

Aims of treatment

Alleviation of symptoms and improvement in quality of life
This is achieved by reducing hyperglycaemia; patients who need insulin immediately (those with Type 1 diabetes) were described in the previous chapter. All others normally begin on diet alone, moving to diet and oral hypoglycaemic agents, or diet and insulin as indicated. All treatments must be adjusted to ensure that patients are symptom-free. Education of patients plays an important role in enhancing the quality of life, and needs to be maintained over many years.

Maintainenance of health by reduction of risk factors and preventing the development of diabetic complications
The needs here are for:

- achievement of optimal blood glucose control
- detection and control of hypertension
- assessment and control of hyperlipidaemia
- assessment of the need for antiplatelet medication
- cessation of smoking
- regular complications screening procedures (described on page 45).

Management of long-term diabetic complications

Management of other medical problems affecting the patient

The aims of controlling diabetes

Once diabetes treatment has been established, there is a need to agree the level of control to be achieved in each individual patient. Once symptoms have been eliminated, targets for optimal control (shown in the table) should be discussed and agreed, but it is not always possible to reach ideal goals and pragmatic decisions have to be made.
    The following criteria need consideration:

- ensure that symptoms have been eliminated
- lean patients should gain weight
- obese patients should lose weight
- children should grow normally
- prevention of long-term diabetic complications.

Healthy lifestyle

People with diabetes can help themselves considerably by attention to healthy eating, appropriate exercise levels and weight reduction, and cessation of smoking. These measures

---

Treatment aims
- Save life
- Alleviate symptoms
- Prevent long-term complications
- Reduce risk factors:
    smoking
    hypertension
    obesity
    hyperlipidaemia
- Educate patients and encourage self-management
- Achieve goals of St Vincent declaration (see page 82)

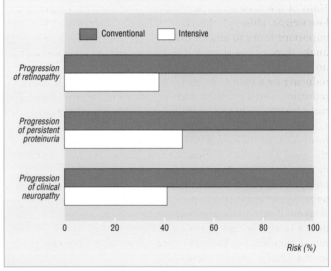

Risk reduction for complications in young Type 1 diabetic patients under intensive diabetic control: results from the DCCT

Targets for control of diabetes

	Very good*	Acceptable	Less than ideal
Body mass index (kg/m^2)	<25	<27	>27
HbA$_{1c}$ (%) (normal 4.0-6.0)	<6.5	6.5-7.5	>7.5 (>8.0 poor)
Blood glucose in Type 2 diabetes† (mmol/l):			
Fasting	<5.5	<8.0	≥10.0
Postprandial	<9.0	<10.0	≥10.0

*This is the ideal and may be difficult, impossible, or unnecessary to achieve in certain patients (for example, elderly people)
Individual targets should be established for each patient
†The optimal range in Type 1 diabetes is about 4.0-9.0 mmol/l

are of great benefit, and may also substantially reduce the need for medication. Behaviour change strategies may be needed to help patients to implement them.

Healthy eating

Healthy eating is the cornerstone of diabetic treatment, and control of the diet should always be the first treatment offered to Type 2 diabetic patients before drugs are considered. Eliminating sugar (sucrose and glucose) lowers blood glucose concentrations in both Type 1 and Type 2 diabetic patients, and although recent dietary recommendations suggest that eating small amounts of sugar is of little consequence, this practice is not recommended. Artificial sweeteners can be used. Good dietary advice is essential to the proper care of diabetic patients; ill considered advice can be very damaging or else it is ignored. I recall one patient who kept to the same sample menu for many years before she reported it to be rather boring. The diet needs to be tailored to the patient's age and weight, type of work, race, and religion.

Recommendations for Type 2 diabetic patients
Diets for overweight Type 2 diabetic patients should aim to eliminate all forms of sugar and restrict the total energy intake. Many of the patients are overweight, and their main goal is to lose weight, although this aim is difficult to achieve. It is important to try to ensure that when patients reduce their intake they do not replace it by an increase of fatty foodstuffs, notably a high intake of cheese. The present emphasis is on reducing total calorie intake, with special emphasis on fat reduction and a proportionately more generous allowance of carbohydrate than in previous years. It has been suggested that as much as half the energy content of the diet may be derived from carbohydrate, while the fat intake is drastically reduced, although these diets in practice require rather difficult and radical changes in the types of food normally eaten. The use of polyunsaturated fats is desirable. These diets are of value and help to reduce blood glucose concentrations if enough fibre is taken. Bran, All Bran, wholemeal bread, and beans have a relatively high fibre content, and are therefore recommended, but foodstuffs with a very high fibre content, such as guar gum, are unpalatable.

For some elderly patients it is enough simply to eliminate all forms of sugar from the diet. Their blood glucose concentrations then fall and symptoms may resolve.

Simple dietary guidelines
- Never take any form of sugar
- Do not take too much fat
- There is no need to restrict most meat, fish, or vegetables
- Control your weight

There is no need to buy proprietary diabetic foodstuffs. Most forms of alcohol (other than sweet wines and liqueurs) are suitable for diabetics, with the usual restrictions for the overweight

A diabetic diet: elimination of sugar/glucose/sucrose
Do not eat or drink:
- Sugar or glucose in any form and do not use sugar in your cooking
- Jam, marmalade, honey, syrup, or lemon curd
- Sweets or chocolates
- Cakes and sweet biscuits
- Tinned fruit
- Lucozade, Ribena, Coca-Cola, Pepsi-Cola, lemonade, or other fizzy drinks

You may use artificial sweeteners, such as saccharin, Sweetex, Hermesetas, Saxin, but NOT Sucron, and any sugar-free drinks including squashes and Slimline range

Fibre content of diet
The following will increase the fibre content of the diet:

Bread	Wholemeal or stoneground— wholemeal for preference If these are not available use HiBran or wheatmeal or granary loaves
Biscuits and crispbreads	Ryvita, Macvita, and similar varieties. Digestive, oatcakes, coconut, and bran biscuits, etc. Crackawheat
Breakfast cereals	Porridge, Weetabix, Weetaflakes, All Bran, Bran Buds, Shredded Wheat, Oat Krunchies, muesli, Alpen, and similar cereals
Wholemeal flour or 100% rye flour	Should be used with white flour for making bread, scones, cakes, biscuits, puddings, etc
Fresh fruit and vegetables	Should be included at least twice daily. The skin and peel of fruit and vegetables such as apples, pears, plums, tomatoes, and potatoes should be eaten
Dried fruit and nuts *Brown rice, wholemeal pasta*	Eat frequently
Pulse vegetables	Such as peas and all varieties of beans

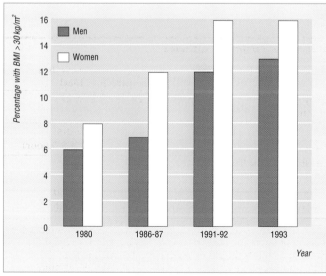

Prevalence of obesity in England

Optimal control may not be needed and it is best to interfere as little as possible with the patient's usual way of life.

Diets for Type 1 diabetic patients
Greater finesse is required in managing the diets of Type 1 diabetic patients; if they eat too much, diabetic control deteriorates; if they eat too little they become hypoglycaemic. The important principles are that carbohydrate intake should be steady from day to day and that it should be taken at fairly regular times each day. If this discipline is not followed diabetic control becomes difficult, although new approaches to the management of Type 1 diabetes such as dose adjustment for normal eating (DAFNE) (see page 29) may permit flexibility in which calculation of carbohydrate intake is used to calculate the insulin dose, thus freeing the patient from a rigidly controlled dietary intake. Severe carbohydrate restriction is not necessarily required; indeed, if the diet is fairly generous patients are less likely to resort to a high fat intake, which may be harmful in the long term.

The actual requirement for carbohydrate varies considerably; it is unsatisfactory to recommend less than 100 g daily, and control may become more difficult if more than 250 g daily is allowed. The smaller amounts are more suitable for elderly, sedentary patients while the larger amounts are more appropriate for younger, very active people particularly athletes who may need considerably more. Although it has been observed that not all carbohydrate-containing foodstuffs are equally absorbed and that they do not have the same influence on blood glucose values, it is impracticable to make allowances for such variations other than recommending that sugar (sucrose) should be avoided except for the treatment of hypoglycaemia.

For social convenience it is customary to advise that most of carbohydrate should be taken at the main meals—breakfast, lunch, and dinner—even though these are not necessarily the times when, according to blood glucose profiles, most carbohydrate is needed; for example, less carbohydrate at breakfast and more at mid-morning and lunch often improves the profile. Snacks should be taken between meals—that is, at elevenses, during the afternoon, and at bedtime—to prevent hypoglycaemia. At least the morning and night snacks are essential and should never be missed.

For the convenience of some, and for those adopting the DAFNE method of controlling Type I diabetes and therefore needing to calculate the carbohydrate content of their meals, 10 g of carbohydrate is described as "one portion" so that a 170 g carbohydrate diet is described to patients as one of "17 portions". Patients sometimes find it valuable to know the carbohydrate values of different foodstuffs.

Foods suitable during intercurrent illness
The presence of malaise, nausea, and anorexia during illness may deter patients from eating, yet food is needed to avoid hypoglycaemia following insulin administration, which should never be stopped (see page 37). Suitable foodstuffs for use at this time are shown in the box.

Weight control: the role of exercise
Weight control towards optimal levels yields considerable health benefits to all, notably in this context to those who have the combined disadvantages of being overweight and having Type 2 diabetes. Exercise has a central role in weight reduction and health improvement. The proven benefits include reduced insulin resistance (hence enhanced insulin sensitivity) leading to better glycaemic control which may even be independent of actual weight reduction. Risk factors for cardiovascular disease,

A sample meal plan for a Type 1 diabetic

	Carbohydrate portions	Recommended food and drink
Breakfast	1	Fruit
	1	Wholemeal cereal
	1	Milk
	1	Wholemeal bread Egg/grilled bacon Tea/coffee
Mid-morning	1	Fruit/plain biscuit Tea/coffee/diet drink
Lunch		Lean meat/fish/ egg/cheese
	2	Potatoes/bread/rice/ pasta
		Vegetable salad
	2	Fruit/sugar-free pudding
Mid-afternoon	1	Fruit/plain biscuit Tea/coffee/diet drink
Dinner		Lean meat/fish/eggs/ cheese
	2	Potatoes/bread/rice/ pasta
		Vegetable salad
	2	Fruit/sugar-free pudding
Bed-time	1	Bread/fruit/plain biscuit Tea/coffee/diet drink
Total 15		

Alcohol
- Alcohols containing simple sugar should not be drunk by people with diabetes, especially sweet wines and liqueurs
- Dry wines and spirits are mainly sugar-free and do not present special problems
- Beers and lagers have a relatively high sugar and calorie content and their amount needs to be both limited and counted as part of the controlled carbohydrate intake
- Sugar-free beers are high in calorie and alcohol content and therefore have some limitations to their usefulness, whereas "low alcohol" beers are high in carbohydrate
- Profound hypoglycaemia may be provoked in those who take large amounts of alcohol, and omit their normal diet, especially in those taking sulphonylureas; this can be dangerous
- Normal social drinking is usually free from this hazard but care is still needed
- Reduction in alcohol intake is sometimes an important part of helping weight loss

Foods suitable during intercurrent illness
For patients who are feeling ill but need to maintain their carbohydrate intake, the following are useful (each item contains 10 g of carbohydrate):
- 1/3 pint (0.15 l) tinned soup
- 1 glass fruit juice
- 1 scoop of ice cream
- 1 glass of milk

The following each contain 20 g of carbohydrate:
- 2 teaspoons Horlicks and milk
- 2 digestive biscuits
- 1 Weetabix and a glass of milk
- 1 ordinary fruit yoghurt
- "Build-up" made with 1/2 a pint (0.25 l) of milk and 1/2 a sachet

which include high blood pressure, also diminish. Indeed, the prevention of Type 2 diabetes itself in those at high risk has been amply demonstrated (see page 6). People with osteoarthritis, chronic heart failure, and chronic lung disease all benefit from appropriate exercise programmes and weight reduction, and there are advantages to those recovering from myocardial infarction. A healthier life is also gained by the very old and by the overweight child. For those with Type 2 diabetes it is recommended that exercise of moderate intensity should be undertaken for about 30 minutes each day. This can include walking, as well as both aerobic and resistance exercise.

The effects of exercise in Type 1 diabetes present the hazard of hypoglycaemia and it is not a specific contributor to improvement of diabetes control. Advice is required on the use of insulin and the need for additional food (in particular carbohydrate) before, during, and after periods of exercise especially (since hypoglycaemia may develop after cessation of exercise) for those engaged in major sports and athletics. The challenge for sportsmen can be extreme but nevertheless people with Type 1 diabetes are known for huge achievements. Great credit went to Sir Steven Redgrave for his ingenious food and insulin regimen which enabled him to win a rowing gold medal in the 2000 Olympic Games.

How 10 fat men and 10 lean men fare on the journey through life (Joslin, 1941)

Smoking

The addiction of smoking is now well established. Its harmful effects are numerous, and include a substantial increase in cardiovascular and peripheral vascular disease as well as the best known consequences of lung cancer and chronic obstructive pulmonary disease. In diabetes, higher rates of both nephropathy and retinopathy have been well documented.

Nicotine replacement therapy using proprietary sublingual preparations, chewing gum, self adhesive patches, or alternatively amfebutamone tablets can help, especially if used in conjunction with the counselling which is provided by smoking clinics. Detailed use of these medications is described in the *British National Formulary* (*BNF*).

The histogram of risk reduction for complication in young Type 1 diabetic patients under intensive diabetic control is adapted from Watkins PJ, et al. *Diabetes and its management*, 5th ed. Oxford: Blackwell Science, 1996.
The histogram showing prevalence of obesity in England is adapted from Nutrition and Obesity Task Force. Obesity: reversing the increasing problems of obesity in England. London: Department of Health, 1995.
The illustration of how 10 fat men and lean men fare through life is from Joslin EP. *Diabetic manual*, 1941, Lea and Febiger.

The story of Mrs B-J continued: the diet

I was put in a Women's ward and I was given my first dose of insulin. The bed was in the centre of the ward and I soon became the ladies' pet. They threw sweets on to my bed, which I politely refused, no doubt recalling how I had forsworn such poison.

I stayed in hospital for three weeks, and each day I was given lessons in diet. I had a red exercise book in which I set out different diets, stating the weight and value of each carbohydrate item. I had a chart with various foods listed. Those printed in black were called "black lines" and had to be limited by weight to equal the "black lines" allowed at each meal. The protein foods were "red lines" and could be taken ad lib.

4   Treatment of Type 2 diabetes mellitus

Type 2 diabetes is a complex disorder generally affecting older people who are often overweight and likely to suffer other medical problems as well. Its management presents considerable challenges to medical and nursing staff, whose care must be directed at the sum of the problems of the individual patient. Management now requires not only attention to blood glucose control, but also to the treatment of hypertension and hyperlipidaemia, as well as introducing the necessary measures for reducing cardiovascular risk factors.

Optimal treatment of Type 2 diabetic patients, especially those who are symptom-free, overweight and have in addition several cardiovascular risk factors, exercises our clinical skills and judgments to the limit. There needs to be a sense of reality within the consultation, bearing in mind the potential dangers of unacceptable polypharmacy accompanied by low adherence to prescribed treatment as well as a sense of guilt experienced by those who fail to achieve ideal targets set by physicians. Awareness of the priorities and intentions of individual patients needs to be given consideration, and patients need to agree on the objectives for treatment. Recommendations for treatment must be clinically relevant for the individual patient, who should be involved in choosing which of the many therapeutic options to select after explanation of advantages and risks. The difficulties of controlling Type 2 diabetes tend to increase with the passage of time as the disease progresses. Management is often difficult and needs to be pragmatic: the late Professor John Malins when asked how this should be done used to quote the advice given by Chekhov to his actors—that it should be "done as well as possible".

> **Approaches to management**
> There are three distinctive aspects in management, each of which requires entirely different approaches
>
> - To alleviate symptoms and improve quality of life, achieved by reducing hyperglycaemia and weight
> - To maintain health by reduction of risk factors (especially hypertension, hyperlipidaemia, and smoking) and by screening programmes to diminish the development of diabetic complications
> - Management of diabetic complications
> - Management of other medical problems

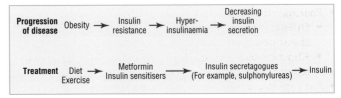

Natural history of Type 2 diabetes

Glycaemic control

Natural history

Type 2 diabetes is an insidiously progressive disease. Gradually decreasing insulin secretion leads to a slow increase in hyperglycaemia and a rise of HbA_{1c} values, often despite vigorous clinical attempts to maintain control. Thus, while control during the early years is often straightforward, it becomes increasingly difficult with the passage of time, so that the appropriate need for tablets and insulin requires continuing consideration.

Non-obese patients
Such patients require different consideration from the obese. They are much more likely to require insulin early in the course of treatment, and indeed apparent presentation as Type 2 diabetes may be deceptive when they progress to Type 1 diabetes as cases of latent autoimmune diabetes of adulthood (LADA). Sulphonylurea treatment is used initially while metformin treatment is inappropriate for these patients. Some of them cling desperately to minute diets with the large doses of sulphonylureas as weight and health decline: these patients regain their health rapidly when insulin treatment is started and indeed it should not be delayed.

Obese patients
These patients require a different approach. The need for healthy eating and exercise in an attempt to reduce weight are paramount yet difficult to achieve. When these measures fail,

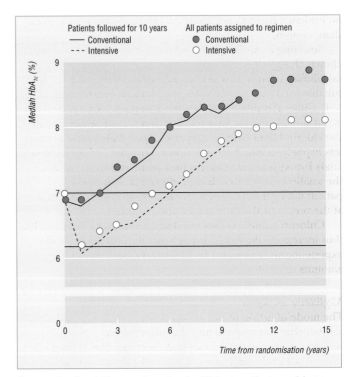

Cross sectional and 10-year cohort data for HbA_{1c} in patients receiving intensive or conventional treatment, from UKPDS (Type 2 diabetes; see page 42)

14

metformin is the first choice, and will to a small extent diminish the weight gain which comes almost inevitably with improved glycaemic control. A sulphonylurea or meglitidine analogue is added when metformin alone fails. The use of thiazolidinediones is described below.

Patients who remain unwell and often symptomatic (thirst and nocturia especially) and who continue to lose weight should be switched to insulin without delay.

Achieving glycaemic control and reducing risk factors
- Healthy lifestyle advice—healthy eating plan, exercise, and weight reduction plan.
- Oral hypoglycaemic agents should be given only when dietary treatment alone has failed after a proper trial period, usually lasting at least three months. They should not normally be given as the initial treatment (this is a common error).
  - **Sulphonylureas** stimulate insulin secretion
  - **Meglitidine analogues** stimulate insulin secretion
  - **Biguanides (metformin)** reduce hepatic gluconeogenesis and enhance glucose uptake
  - **Thiazolidinediones** enhance insulin sensitivity
  - **α glucosidase inhibitors (acarbose)** reduce absorption of complex carbohydrates.
- Pharmacological agents to assist weight reduction:
  - **Orlistat** inhibits pancreatic lipase and reduces fat absorption
  - **Sibutramine** is a monoamine reuptake inhibitor, causing reduced appetite
- Antihypertensive and lipid lowering agents (see chapter 17).

Sulphonylureas
Seven sulphonylureas are available. They are remarkably safe and free from side effects, although rare toxic effects have been reported, including rashes and jaundice. Only one sulphonylurea should be used at a time since there is nothing to be gained from any combination of these drugs and there is no evidence that any one drug is likely to be more successful than another.

Selecting a sulphonylurea is largely a matter of personal choice, though it is now usual to use one of the shorter acting, metabolised drugs such as gliclazide or glipizide, which are suitable for all ages and for those with renal impairment as well. Glibenclamide, which has the advantage of once-daily use, is still suitable for younger patients, but is contraindicated in the elderly. Glimepiride is also given once daily and may cause less hypoglycaemia. Excessive doses can cause hazardous (even fatal) hypoglycaemia, and it is thus usual to start treatment with the smallest useful dose. If hypoglycaemia does occur in a patient taking a sulphonylurea, the drug should be stopped or at the very least the dose substantially reduced.

Chlorpropamide is now obsolete. It has a very long half life, thus increasing the risk of hypoglycaemia, and many patients experience an unpleasant facial flush on drinking very small amounts of alcohol.

Meglitidine analogues
The mode of action of this group of drugs is similar to that of sulphonylureas though acting at a different site. Their advantages are the rapid onset and short half life, efficacy when taken just 15 minutes before meals, and a duration of effect of no more than three hours. They are omitted if no meal is taken. There may be some benefit in reducing postprandial glycaemia and in theory at least there might be less hypoglycaemia.

Daily dose ranges for oral hypoglycaemic agents

Oral hypoglycaemic agents	Dose range (mg)
Sulphonylureas	
Glibenclamide (×1/day)	2·5-15
Gliclazide	40-320
Glimepiride (×1/day)	1-4
Glipizide	2·5-20
Gliquidone	15-180
Tolbutamide	500-2000
*Meglitidine analogues**	
Nateglinide	180-540
Repaglinide	1·5-16
Biguanide	
Metformin	1000-2000
Thiazolidinediones	
Pioglitazone (×1/day)	15-30
Rosiglitazone	4-8
α *glucosidase inhibitors*	
Acarbose	50-600

*Meglitidine analogues are taken three times daily; before meals. Most of the other drugs can be started as single daily doses, but as requirements increase are more effective in divided doses

The hypoglycaemic effect of early sulphonamides was observed in the 1940s, and in the next decade first tolbutamide (1956) and then chlorpropamide (1957) were introduced into clinical practice. They act chiefly by stimulating insulin release from the B-cells of pancreatic islets

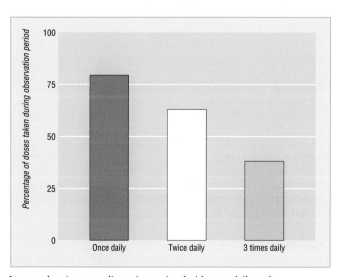

Increased patient compliance is associated with once-daily oral hypoglycaemic agents

Nateglinide is one of a new class of oral hypoglycaemic agents, namely an amino acid derivative. Insulin release after meals is both faster and of shorter duration than that with either sulphonylureas or repaglinide, giving less postprandial hyper-insulinaemia and less reactive hypoglycaemia. It is licensed only for use in combination with metformin, but not for monotherapy or substitution for conventional sulphonylureas.

Biguanides: metformin
Biguanides act chiefly by reducing hepatic glucose production. They also enhance peripheral glucose uptake, and to some extent reduce carbohydrate absorption. Metformin is the only biguanide available in the United Kingdom. It is the drug of choice in the treatment of overweight Type 2 diabetic patients when diet alone has failed. UKPDS found some evidence for a reduction in mortality after the use of metformin.

Lactic acidosis is a serious consequence of the inappropriate use of metformin. It is contraindicated in any patient with renal failure, and serum creatinine should be monitored. A creatinine concentration above 150 μmol/l indicates that the drug should be stopped. Metformin should not be used in any seriously ill or shocked patient, nor in those with heart failure, serious liver disease or a very high alcohol intake. It is not appropriate for the treatment of thin diabetic patients nor for use in frail elderly patients.

α Glucosidase inhibitors
These agents block the enzyme responsible for the breakdown of complex carbohydrates in the gut and can effectively reduce the increase in blood glucose after a meal. Acarbose acts in this way and can be used alone or in combination with other oral hypoglycaemic agents. Its hypoglycaemic effect is relatively small and the severe flatulence which develops (to some extent avoidable by starting with small amounts) deters many patients from using it.

Thiazolidinediones
This newly introduced group of hypoglycaemic agents act by reducing insulin resistance and by activation of the peroxisome proliferator activated receptor γ expressed predominantly in adipose tissue.

These drugs are licensed for use with metformin if this alone has failed to control the diabetes, or with a sulphonylurea if metformin is either not tolerated or contraindicated (for example, in renal failure). In the European Union they are not licensed for use alone or in combination with insulin, and should not be given to patients with a history of heart failure, or during pregnancy. They may cause oedema, a minor reduction of haemoglobin, and a small increase of HDL cholesterol. There are very rare reports of liver dysfunction, and liver function should be monitored before, and every two months after, starting treatment, for the following 12 months.

Drugs for management of obesity
There is a limited place for the use of medication in assisting with weight reduction in the obese diabetic patient. The use of such drugs is restricted to those whose BMI is 28 or more and who are between the ages of 18 and 65 years; they should only be prescribed for individuals who have lost at least 2·5 kg body weight by diet and exercise during the preceding month. Patients should continue to be supported by their advisers and counsellors throughout treatment. Orlistat inhibits fat absorption by inhibition of pancreatic lipase. Weight reduction

Use of metformin
- Drug of first choice for overweight Type 2 diabetes
- May reduce mortality (UKPDS)
- Never use when creatinine is >150 μmol/l
- Danger of lactic acidosis if given to:
  renal failure patients
  patients with liver disease
  patients with a high alcohol intake
- Not to be used for thin patients or those in heart failure
- During intravenous contrast procedures:
  stop metformin for 48 hours beforehand and do not restart until 48 hours after procedure completed

Side effects of metformin
- Nausea
- Diarrhoea
- Metallic taste

These effects can be minimised by starting with a low dose and taking tablets during meals. The effects generally resolve with time

Thiazolidinediones should be used in patients expected to be insulin resistant, namely those who are overweight and likely to be hyperlipidaemic and hypertensive as well

Useful drug combinations
- Sulphonylurea (or metaglitidine analogue) with metformin
- Sulphonylurea (or metaglinide analogue) with thiazolidinedione (if metformin is contraindicated or not tolerated)
- Metformin with thiazolidinedione
- Nateglinide with metformin
- Metformin with insulin (for overweight patients)
- Acarbose can be used in association with any of the above

indicating a successful response should be greater than 5% after 12 weeks, in which event prescription may be continued for one year to a limit of two years, otherwise treatment should cease. Unpleasant oily leakage and steatorrhoea can occur.

Sibutramine also acts centrally as a serotonin and noradrenaline reuptake inhibitor and enhances the satiety response. It is used as an adjunct to weight maintenance after weight loss. Full details of its use and contraindications are to be found in the *BNF*.

Guar gum
Guar gum preparations, taken in adequate quantity three times daily before meals, can reduce postprandial blood glucose concentrations. Flatulence is common and often unacceptable. Guarem is the only available preparation. It has a very limited role.

Hypoglycaemia
Only sulphonylureas and meglitidine analogues cause hypoglycaemia, but it should not be allowed to occur at all—it almost invariably indicates excessive dosage. Those most at risk are elderly people who may make dosage errors or fail to take their normal meals. Hypoglycaemia in this situation can be fatal. The shorter acting sulphonylureas cause the least hypoglycaemia and are therefore best for older people (see below). Management of hypoglycaemia is described in chapter 8. β Blockers may not only exacerbate hypoglycaemia, but also occasionally inhibit the early warning symptoms.

Indications for insulin in Type 2 diabetes
Approximately 6% of non-obese and 2% of obese Type 2 diabetic patients need to start insulin each year. Predicting the need for insulin is difficult: those of lean body mass, especially in the presence of islet cell antibodies, are at greatest risk.

Whether to give insulin to Type 2 diabetic patients is one of the most important yet difficult decisions to be made in treating these patients. Failure to give insulin to some patients results in protracted and needless malaise if not actual danger. On the other hand, giving insulin inappropriately can cause needless problems, notably from hypoglycaemia and weight gain.

Indications for giving insulin to Type 2 diabetic patients who are inadequately controlled despite adherence to their recommended diet and oral hypoglycaemic agents are as follows:

- Continuing weight loss (even if this is insidious), and persistent symptoms, or both. Insulin treatment in these patients almost always results in a substantial improvement in health.
- A non-obese patient without symptoms whose weight is stable and who is conscientious with existing medication. Diabetic control will usually improve, and about half of the patients will enjoy an improvement in well-being.
- An obese patient without symptoms whose weight is stable presents an even more difficult problem. The correct management is to ensure that they are taking their medication, together with intensification of diet, but sometimes insulin may be needed simply to improve control of diabetes in order to reduce long-term complications during the following decade or more. A reduction of HbA$_{1C}$ of approximately 2% together with weight gain of around 5-7 kg can be expected. Unfortunately improvement in glycaemic control is not always achieved. Patient choice is important here, and some prefer not to take insulin after all explanations have been presented. Reluctant patients can be

Drug interactions
- Alcohol can cause serious hypoglycaemia when used with sulphonureas and lactic acidosis in those taking metformin
- Aspirin, sulphonamides, and monoamine oxidase inhibitors may enhance the hypoglycaemic action of sulphonylureas, but in practice problems are rarely seen
- Selective serotonin reuptake inhibitors used in the treatment of depression may provoke hypoglycaemia
- Serious hyperglycaemia is provoked by corticosteroids, dopexamine (inotropic support agent) and intravenous β agonists (salbutamol, terbutaline, ritrodrine)
- Thiazide diuretics (other than minimum dosage, for example, bendrofluazide 2·5 mg) can exacerbate hyperglycaemia
- The immunosuppressive drug ciclosporin can also exacerbate hyperglycaemia
- Protease inhibitors used in the treatment of patients with HIV can cause a syndrome of lipodystrophy, hyperlipidaemia, and insulin resistance leading to severe exacerbation of hyperglycaemia or even causing diabetes
- Clozapine may provoke hyperglycaemia
- β blockers may exacerbate hyperglycaemia or hypoglycaemia depending on dose, concomitant medication, nutritional state, severity of illness, and the patient's age
- Other less common drug interactions are described in the *BNF*

Indications for insulin in Type 2 diabetes
- Insulin is usually contraindicated in overweight patients whose weight is increasing—giving insulin will make this worse
- Patients who continue to lose weight usually need insulin
- Achievement of tight control in order to prevent complications is obviously more appropiate in younger than in older patients, so the patient's age needs to be considered in deciding whether or not to start giving insulin
- Many older patients, however, benefit greatly from insulin treatment, with an improvement of well-being, and insulin should not be withheld on grounds of age alone

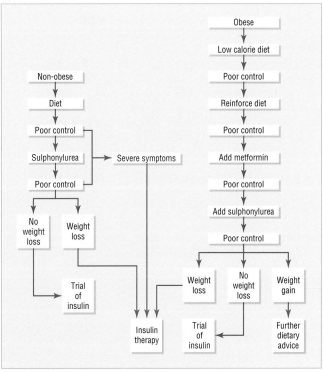

Indications for insulin in Type 2 diabetes mellitus

given a three-month trial of insulin and then make their decision, which experience shows to be usually affirmative. Those with a short life expectancy do not necessarily benefit, and those with other medical disorders will require individual consideration.

- Insulin is often required in patients with intercurrent illness. Many disorders, notably infections, increase insulin resistance, leading to the temporary need for insulin. Withdrawal of insulin after recovering from the illness is important provided adequate control is achieved and maintained.

Corticosteroids always exacerbate hyperglycaemia and often precipitate the need for insulin. This should not deter doctors from prescribing them when they are needed.

Combination treatment with insulin and metformin

Metformin can be given together with insulin to overweight Type 2 diabetic patients: this can to a small extent limit the inevitable weight gain following introduction of insulin. A combination of sulphonylureas with insulin gives little benefit and has the added disadvantage that patients must continue with both modes of treatment.

Insulin regimens suitable for Type 2 diabetic patients are described in chapter 5.

The figure showing the cross sectional and 10-year cohort data for HbA_{1c} in patients receiving intensive or conventional treatment is adapted from UKPDS *Lancet* 1998;352:837-53 with permission from Elsevier Science. The histogram showing increased patient compliance is adapted from Paes AH, Bakker AS, Soe Agnie CJ. Impact of dosage frequency upon patient compliance. *Diabetes Care* 1997;20:1512-17.

5   Insulin treatment

I was like a dried tree, but you have given me new life.
                    An Ethiopian villager, after starting insulin.

The astonishing power of insulin to restore health and well-being to rapidly deteriorating newly diagnosed Type 1 diabetic patients is as remarkable now as it was in 1922. After Banting gave insulin to Elizabeth Hughes in that year, she wrote to her mother that "it is simply too wonderful for words this stuff." Insulin to this day always has this effect; the challenge now is to optimise control in order to maintain health throughout life.

Insulin is also needed to enhance well-being and control in many Type 2 diabetic patients when the natural progression of their disease has lead to loss of optimal control. The potential to reduce the development of long-term diabetic complications as demonstrated by the UKPDS (see page 42) has led to a recent explosion in conversions from tablets to insulin. The difficult decisions which surround the need for insulin in this situation, together with benefits, uses and misuses of insulin have been described in the previous chapter.

The use of insulin must be tailored to meet individual requirements. The aim is to achieve the best possible control in the circumstances, avoiding at all costs the disabling hypoglycaemia which can occur if control is excessively tight. In some elderly patients and those who lack motivation, it is therefore wise to aim only at alleviating symptoms and not to attempt very strict control.

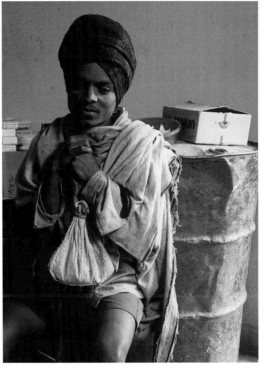

An Ethiopian patient carrying his diabetes equipment to the clinic

Types of insulin

Soluble insulins
These were first introduced in 1922. They have a rapid onset of action (within 15-30 minutes) and a relatively short overall duration of action of six to eight hours. They play an important part in both daily maintenance of diabetic patients by subcutaneous injection, and also in managing emergencies, when they can be given intravenously or intramuscularly. Other insulin preparations are not suitable for intravenous or intramuscular use.

New recombinant insulin analogues
These have a very rapid onset and very short action, and have been developed by altering the structure and thus the property of the insulin. The preparations available in the United Kingdom

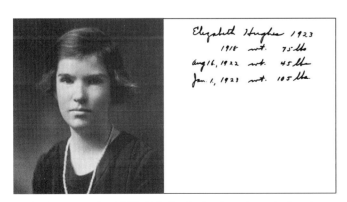

Elizabeth Evans Hughes (1907-1981). Banting's prize patient, who found insulin "unspeakably wonderful." The photograph is from Banting's scrapbook

Insulins available in the United Kingdom
Insulins are available as human, pork or beef preparations, or as insulin analogues.

Very short acting insulin analogues
- Insulin Aspart (Novo Rapid)
- Insulin Lispro (Humalog)

Short acting neutral soluble insulins
- Human Actrapid
- Human Velosulin
- Humulin S
- Insuman Rapid
- Pork Actrapid
- Pork Neutral
- Beef Neutral

Medium acting isophane insulins
- Human Insulatard
- Humulin I
- Insuman Basal
- Pork Insulatard
- Pork Isophane
- Beef Isophane

Medium acting insulin zinc suspensions
- Human Monotard
- Humulin Lente
- Lentard MC (beef or pork)
- Beef Lente

Long acting insulin zinc suspensions
- Human Ultratard
- Humulin Zinc

Long acting insulin analogue
- Insulin Glargine

at present are Insulin Lispro (Humalog) and Insulin Aspart (Novo Rapid). They have some advantages because they may be given immediately before meals (or even immediately after meals if necessary). By virtue of their very short action, there is less hypoglycaemia before the next meal, and when they are used before the main evening meal nocturnal hypoglycaemia is effectively reduced.

There is a risk of postprandial hypoglycaemia if they are used before a meal with a very high fat content because of the delayed gastric emptying. Duration of action is short and does not normally exceed three hours, and their use is therefore inappropriate if the gap between meals exceeds about four hours. Preprandial blood glucose levels are slightly higher than with conventional soluble insulins.

They are also ideal for use in continuous subcutaneous insulin infusion pumps (CSII).

Protamine insulins
These are medium duration insulins introduced in Denmark during the 1930s. Isophane insulin is the most frequently used insulin in this group.

Insulin zinc suspensions
These were first introduced during the 1950s; there are several preparations with widely ranging durations of action. There are limited indications for using insulins with a very long duration of action (ultratard).

Insulin glargine
This is a new prolonged action, soluble insulin analogue (clear solution) forming a microprecipitate after subcutaneous injection. Its onset of action is after about 90 minutes, it has a prolonged plateau rather than a peak, and lasts 24 hours or more. Thus it mimics more closely the basal insulin secretion of healthy people. When taken at bedtime it reduces the incidence of nocturnal hypoglycaemia, and also reduces the prebreakfast hyperglycaemia. It does not appear to reduce symptomatic or severe hypoglycaemia during the day, and there is no significant beneficial effect on overall diabetic control. More extensive clinical experience in using this insulin is still needed.

Insulin mixtures
Some preparations of insulin are presented as proprietary mixtures in either vials or pen cartridges, eliminating the need for patients to mix insulins in the syringe. The most popular mixture contains 30% soluble insulin and 70% isophane, whereas the whole range also includes ratios 10%/90%, 20%/80%, 40%/60%, and 50%/50%. These insulin mixtures represent a considerable advantage for many patients, especially those who find it difficult to mix insulins in the syringe or those whose visual acuity is impaired. Details of the types of insulin available in the United Kingdom are shown in the box.

Selection of insulin

The choice of insulin preparation is based on the duration of action. Although insulins can be broadly classified as having very short, short, medium or long duration of action, their effect varies considerably from one patient to another and can be discovered in the individual patient only by trial and error. There are several preparations of medium acting insulins, but those most often used are either one of the isophane preparations or less frequently Human Monotard zinc insulin preparation (see box on page 19).

Most patients (85%) now use insulin of human sequence, a few prefer porcine preparations, while use of some insulin

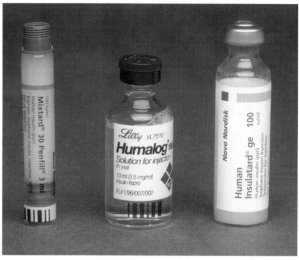

Some insulins

Insulin mixtures
These are all mixtures of a short acting soluble insulin (or very short acting insulin analogue) with a medium acting isophane insulin (or insulin analogue). The number after the insulin name indicates the percentage of the short acting insulin, for example, "30" or "M3" indicates 30% soluble insulin mixed with 70% isophane insulin.

- Human Mixtard 10 (pen only)
- Human Mixtard 20 (pen only)
- Humulin M2 (pen only)
- Human Mixtard 30
- Humulin M3
- Human Mixtard 40 (pen only)
- Human Mixtard 50
- Humulin M5
- Insuman Comb 50
- Insuman Comb 15
- Insuman Comb 25

- Pork Mixtard 30
- Pork 30/70 Mix

Insulin analogue mixtures
- Humalog Mix 25 (pen only)
- Humalog Mix 50 (pen only)
- NovoMix 30 (pen only)

Insulins are available in vials for use with syringe and needle; in cartridges for use in insulin pens; or in preloaded pens. The insulins listed above are available in one or more of these preparations.

analogues with specific indications is increasing (see also chapters 6 and 8). Some preparations of bovine insulins are still available for the few patients who prefer them.

Insulin regimens

Starting insulin in patients with Type 1 diabetes

Some patients start treatment with twice-daily insulin injections using either a mixture containing premixed short and medium acting insulins twice daily or medium acting insulin alone; 8 units twice daily, 15 to 30 minutes before meals is a suitable initial dose for most patients; others will start with a three or four times daily regimen. Only those who are seriously weakened or ill need hospital admission and treatment either with intravenous insulin and fluids or multiple insulin injections. Many patients who present with acute diabetes enter partial remission soon after diagnosis, known as the "honeymoon" phase, when a small dose of almost any insulin is enough to maintain control. The practice of withdrawing insulin at this stage is not encouraged because after a few months the need for insulin is almost inevitable.

Maintenance regimens

Most Type 1 diabetic patients who want to achieve very good control will need at least thrice-daily injections. Multiple injections (three or four times daily) may improve control, reduce the risk of serious hypoglycaemia, and to some extent increase flexibility (for example, the timing of the midday meal) and are often needed in pregnancy. Suitable insulin regimens are as follows:

Twice daily: short and medium acting insulins or occasionally medium acting insulin alone are taken twice daily before breakfast and the main evening meal.

Three times daily: the mixture of neutral soluble and medium acting insulins is taken before breakfast; neutral soluble insulin alone before the evening meal; medium acting insulin alone before bedtime. This insulin regimen has the advantage that the noon injection is not required and is thus favoured by many. Fasting blood glucose is also improved using this regimen.

Four times daily: neutral soluble insulin alone or a short acting insulin analogue is taken before each of the three main meals, and medium acting insulin at bedtime. (Occasionally the long acting Human Ultratard insulin is used, though this has not proved to be as advantageous as it should be in theory.) Sometimes there is a further advantage in adding a medium acting insulin to the prebreakfast soluble insulin.

For some Type 2 diabetic patients, when control on oral medication fails, a single daily injection may suffice; the use of medium acting insulin at bedtime alone has gained popularity and by lowering fasting blood glucose may achieve an acceptable profile throughout the day. This regimen can be usefully combined with concurrent use of metformin. If this fails, insulin needs to be delivered on a twice daily basis or more often, as described above. Premixed insulin mixtures are valuable for many Type 2 diabetic patients.

When changing from one insulin regimen to another some trial and error by regular blood glucose monitoring is always needed. In converting a patient to the four times daily regimen the normal dose should be divided by four and a slight adjustment made to give more than one-quarter before breakfast and less than one-quarter before bedtime.

Administration of insulin

Insulin "pens" and syringes

The use of insulin "pen" devices which deliver metered doses of insulin from an insulin cartridge is now favoured by most

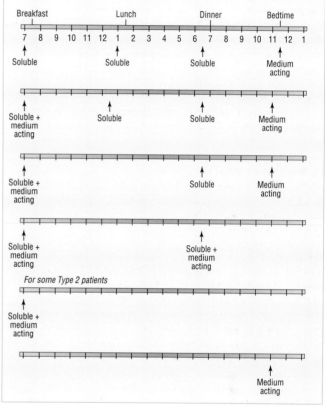

Insulin regimens: short acting insulin analogues can replace conventional soluble insulins

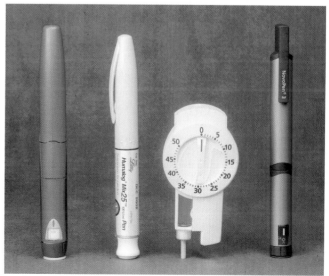

Examples of insulin pens

patients. They are portable and simplify the procedure of measuring the insulin dose. The required dose can be dialled, and some pens feature audible and palpable dose graduations which are of value to those with impaired vision. Some versions of the pen are preloaded and disposable.

Plastic insulin syringes with needle attached are still preferred by some patients, and they are still required by those who prefer to mix individual insulins in the syringe. They can be reused several times and between use can be stored in a refrigerator.

Insulin pumps
Sophisticated insulin pumps infuse insulin subcutaneously over 24 hours, with facilities for preprandial boosts. They are worn on a belt and attached to a subcutaneous cannula. They are expensive and not at present available on the NHS although they should be. They are of value for selected patients with Type 1 diabetes. For more detail regarding their use, see page 29.

Inhaled insulin
While nasal administration of insulin proved unsuccessful, the use of inhaled insulin looks promising. Absorption though inefficient is adequate to reduce hyperglycaemia, and this route of administration may prove to be of value, notably in Type 2 diabetic patients. The practicality of this technique is still under investigation.

Pancreas transplantation
For those needing a kidney transplantation, pancreas transplantation can be performed simultaneously, eliminating the need for insulin injections and rendering glucose tolerance normal or very nearly normal. Five years after transplantation, 60% of patients remain well without needing insulin injections (see page 70).

Islet cell transplantation
The feasibility of islet transplantation has been demonstrated, and with novel immunosuppression techniques islet survival has improved considerably, eliminating the need for injected insulin over increasing periods of time up to three years. Intensive research of this technique is in progress, and at present it is only available for those participating in carefully organised research trials now conducted in several centres including some in the United Kingdom.

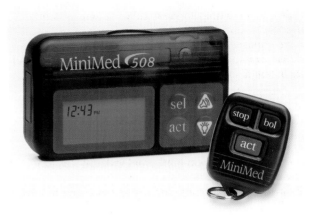

Insulin pump

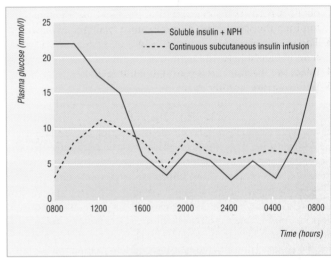

Effect of continuous subcutaneous insulin infusion on plasma glucose

Insulin injection sites

Insulin for routine treatment is given subcutaneously by intermittent injections or by continuous infusion. Insulin can be injected subcutaneously almost anywhere if there is enough flesh. The best site is the front of the thigh. The lower abdominal wall, buttocks, and upper arms may also be used. Patients who want to wear sleeveless clothes should normally avoid using the arms in case unsightly marks or fat hypertrophy should appear; some may then prefer to confine injections to the lower abdomen.

It is important to vary the injection sites from day to day, using for example, each thigh alternately over as wide an area as possible. Absorption of insulin varies from one site to another, being most rapid from the abdominal site, and less rapid from the arms and least from the legs. If there are any difficulties with "control" it is advisable to use one area consistently—for example, the thigh.

In diabetic emergencies soluble insulin is given intravenously, or occasionally intramuscularly (see chapter 9).

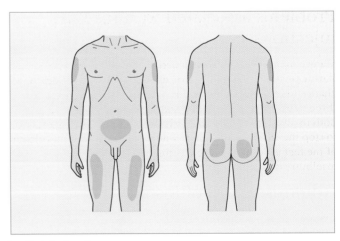

Insulin injection sites

Injection of insulin

Drawing up insulin from the vials

1 Clean the top of the insulin bottle with industrial methylated spirit.
2 Draw air into the syringe to the number of units of insulin required and inject this into the insulin bottle.
3 Draw the required dose of insulin into the syringe, and before withdrawing the needle from the insulin bottle, expel the air bubble if one has formed.

   If clear and cloudy insulins are to be mixed:

1 Inject the correct number of units of air first into the cloudy insulin bottle.
2 Withdraw the needle from the cloudy bottle.
3 Inject the air into the clear bottle, and withdraw the insulin into the syringe.
4 Finally, insert the needle into the cloudy bottle and withdraw the insulin.

Injecting insulin

1 The skin needs to be clean, but application of spirit, which hardens the skin, is not necessary.
2 Stretching the skin at the injection site is the best way to obtain a painless injection; in thin people it may be necessary to pinch the skin between thumb and forefinger of the hand.
3 The needle should be inserted briskly at 90 degrees to the skin, to its whole length.
4 Inject the insulin by depressing the plunger.
5 Withdraw the needle briskly.

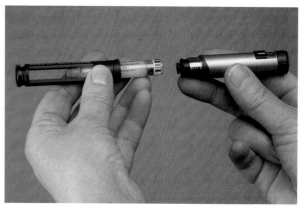
Loading insulin cartridge into pen

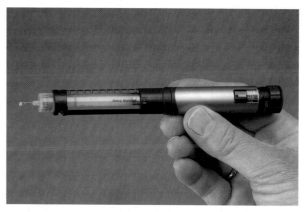
Checking dose and expelling the air

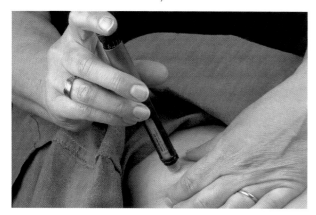
Depressing the plunger

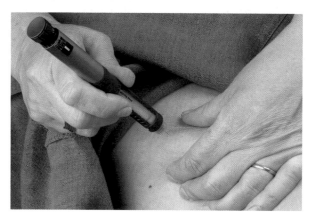
Inserting the needle

Problems associated with insulin injections

Many patients develop some blurring of vision soon after starting insulin, which makes reading difficult. This is due to a change of lens refraction, and it corrects itself within two to three weeks. Patients should be advised that this may occur, both to avoid extreme anxiety which they may experience, and to stop the needless purchase of new glasses. Transient oedema of the feet is not uncommon during the first few weeks of insulin treatment.

Fatty lumps at injection sites are common, and occasionally so large as to be unsightly. Their cause is not known but they sometimes develop if injections are repeatedly given over a very limited area of skin. For this reason it is best to vary the site from day to day. They are rarely troublesome, but once present they tend to persist; the occasional very large fatty tumour may even require surgical removal. Furthermore if insulin is repeatedly injected into a fatty lump, the rate of absorption may be delayed and this may have some adverse effect on blood glucose control. Fat atrophy at injection sites is now very rare.

Red itchy marks at injection sites after starting insulin are also rare, and if they do occur usually disappear spontaneously. If they are very troublesome, adding hydrocortisone to the insulin bottle so that each dose contains about 1 mg eliminates the problem. Insulin allergy causing urticaria still occurs from time to time though it is certainly a very infrequent event: investigation by skin testing and desensitisation may be needed. Abscesses at injection sites are also remarkably rare.

The illustration of Elizabeth Evans Hughes is from Bliss M. *The discovery of insulin.* Edinburgh: Paul Harris, 1983. The photographs of insulin pens and insulin pump are published with permission from Eli Lilly, Novo Nordisk, and Medtronic MiniMed Ltd.

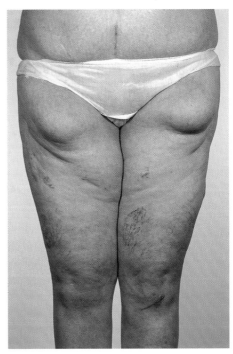

Fatty lumps at injection sites

The story of Mrs B-J continued: starting insulin

I was put in a Women's ward where I was given my first dose of insulin. I can remember vividly my parents' first visit and my mother's anxious face as she walked down the ward, with one enormous white chrysanthemum in her hand. She had expected to see me prone and white and half dead, not sitting up and a picture of health.

I had a lesson on how insulin burnt up the sugar and produced energy, so that I could return to my former activities, and before long I was doing my own injections. I stayed in hospital for three weeks. The Sunday before I was discharged, my parents were asked to come to the diabetic kitchen to witness me doing my insulin and explaining what I was eating and how it had to be calculated. My mother did not see the injection, having passed out, and she told Sister Wheeler that she would never understand the diet. Sister replied "Don't worry about it. She knows, so give her what she tells you". Such confidence was well founded, as my mother never got the hang of it, and I used to write out the amount of potato etc. before I went to school, and my mother would weigh it up before serving it.

They bought all the necessary equipment from King's when I was discharged, including a very solid metal syringe case which I used constantly until it became redundant with the advent of U100 insulin, and also a copy of RD Lawrence's book "A Diabetic ABC". I also had a marvellous pair of German-made scales which would weigh up to 2lbs."

6 Blood glucose monitoring: optimising diabetic control

There are two important reasons for optimising diabetes control: the first is to eliminate symptoms, and the second is the longer-term aim of aborting the development of diabetic complications. Before embarking on complex programmes, it is essential to have a clear view of the requirements of each individual patient. The malaise associated with poorly controlled diabetes almost always responds to better treatment with considerable improvement in well-being. Occasionally, those whose control has been persistently poor for very long periods may for a time feel less well when blood glucose levels are reduced and consequently are at first reluctant to make the effort to improve control.

> The key to achieving optimal diabetes control is regular blood glucose measurement accompanied by a clear understanding of the diurnal profiles so obtained. The optimal insulin regimen can then be devised

Blood glucose measurement

Equipment
- A spring-loaded finger pricking device.
- A blood glucose meter and test strips.
- For some, a blood ketone meter combined with a blood glucose meter and test strips.

   Note: The MiniMed Continuous Glucose Monitoring System measures interstitial glucose levels every 10 seconds using a sensor inserted under the skin of the abdominal wall; and Glucowatch worn on the wrist is a new technique which repeatedly measures subcutaneous glucose levels. They are still expensive, and more experience in ascertaining their reliability is needed before recommending them for routine use.

Purpose
- Spot check to detect hypoglycaemia or impending hypoglycaemia.
- Assess control at times of illness.
- Assess blood glucose profile over 24 hours in order to achieve ideal diabetic control.

   Apart from the first two indications, isolated blood glucose readings are of little value for optimising control.

Timing and frequency of testing for blood glucose profiles for Type 1 diabetes
- One or two tests should be performed each day as a routine for stable patients.
- Tests should be done at different time points each day to build up a profile over several weeks (see page 27).
- A 12-hour profile can be measured on a single day from time to time, taking recordings before meals (four times a day), one to two hours after meals (three times a day) and at bedtime. Occasionally it helps to record a reading around 3 am.

Detecting and eliminating hypoglycaemia (see also chapter 8)
Measurement of blood glucose by patients themselves, or by their relatives, when hypoglycaemia is suspected is the only way of establishing whether or not the blood glucose is actually low. This is of particular value in the assessment of children during periods of bad behaviour, unconsciousness or convulsions. Prediction of hypoglycaemia and therefore prevention is also valuable especially at vulnerable times, notably mid-morning, and at bedtime. Methods of reducing the risks of hypoglycaemia are described in chapters 5 and 8.

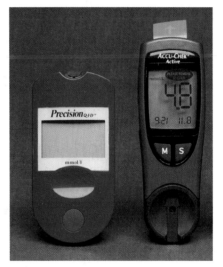

Some blood glucose meters

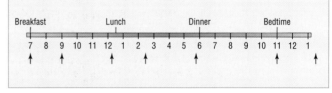

Times for taking blood

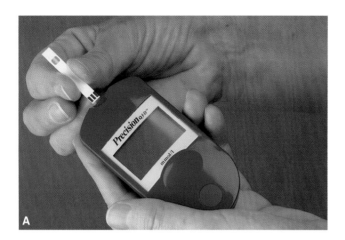

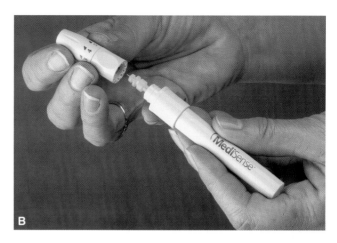

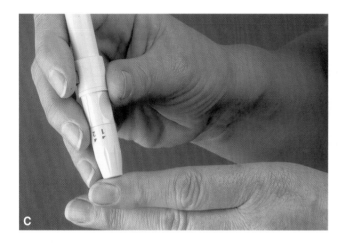

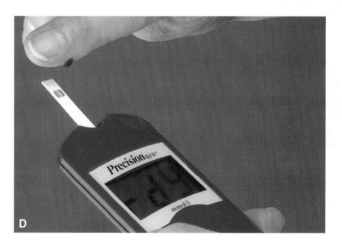

Blood glucose profiles

Assessment by insulin-treated patients of the daily fluctuations of their blood glucose values gives a much greater understanding by patients and doctors of both diabetic control and the effects of different insulin preparations. Indeed, home blood glucose measurement provides an important educational exercise for all seriously motivated diabetic patients as well as being the essential tool to achieve tight blood glucose control. Reproducible blood glucose profiles are essential for making rational adjustments to treatment. They can show not only the times of the peaks and troughs of blood glucose concentration but also the duration of action of different insulin preparations in an individual patient. Unfortunately, those whose lifestyles are chaotic also produce chaotic blood glucose profiles.

Home blood glucose monitoring by the correct technique, combined with the ability to understand the true significance of the readings, represents on the one hand a very important aspect of diabetes care. On the other hand, obsessional patients who perform tests too often with frequent alterations of insulin dose, cause themselves protracted misery and often disabling hypoglycaemia. While this approach sometimes evolves as a result of the patient's personality, such techniques are all too often encouraged by medical attendants.

The aim is to maintain blood glucose in an acceptable range, usually about 4·5 to 7·7 mmol/l before meals, 6·0-9·0 mmol/l after meals, and >7·0-9·0 mmol/l at bedtime.

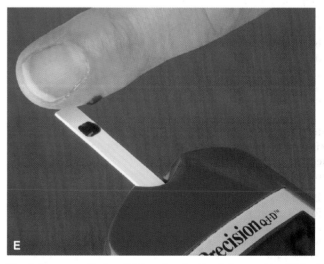

Blood glucose monitoring. (A) Inserting the blood glucose strip; (B) loading the finger pricker; (C) pricking the finger; (D) applying the blood to the testing strip; and (E) awaiting result

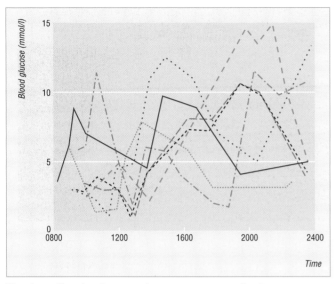

Chaotic profiles taken by one patient on seven consecutive days

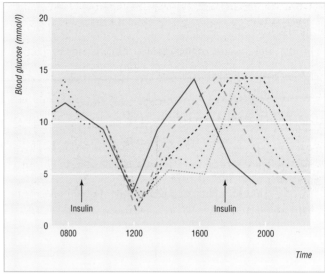

Reproducible profiles taken by one patient on five consecutive days

Occasional excursions outside this range are inevitable, leading to either transient hypoglycaemia or equally transient hyperglycaemia. Thus the occasional high blood glucose readings in an otherwise satisfactory profile can be ignored, although patients are strongly advised to avoid readings below 4·0 mmol/l which if frequent can lead to impaired warning symptoms of hypoglycaemia.

Patients should not respond to isolated high blood glucose readings by taking extra insulin: this causes worsening of blood glucose oscillations rather than an improvement in their blood glucose profile.

Preparing blood glucose profiles
- From patients' record books: visual scanning of records can often detect times of peak and trough readings. Some patients plot their readings graphically which can be very helpful. A few patients present spurious readings which may be difficult to detect.
- Computer-generated profiles: memory records from some blood glucose meters can be downloaded using specially designed computer programs. They can show an excellent visual presentation of readings of any selected time period and may clearly delineate peaks and troughs through 24 hours. Some meters offer this programme on an inbuilt screen.

Interpretation of blood glucose profiles
Before adjusting insulin treatment, it is essential to understand the causes of fluctuating patterns of the blood glucose profile through 24 hours. The following points are crucial.

- Blood glucose rises as insulin action declines, even when no food is taken, because of hepatic gluconeogenesis. This accounts especially for the rapid increase in blood glucose which occurs in the small hours of the morning *before* breakfast.
- These rapid changes in blood glucose also explain why so many patients record different blood glucose readings each day, since even a half to one hour difference in timing can give a very different result.
- Troughs in the blood glucose profile—that is, representing a tendency to hypoglycaemia—almost always occur around noon and between 3 and 5 am at peak insulin activity, so that measures need to be taken to avoid hypoglycaemia especially preceding these times.

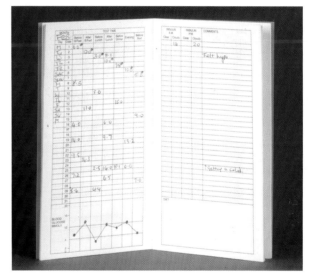

Blood glucose recording book

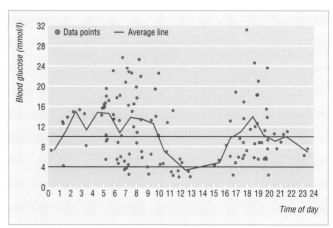

Computer-generated blood glucose profile. Modal day—data points with average line. Patient tends to measure blood glucose at extremes. Target range: high 10.0, low 4.0

- When patients perform three or four isolated blood glucose readings over 24 hours, it is essential for them and their advisers to understand what happens to the blood glucose profile between the single readings. Thus, readings taken at points A, B, C, and D give a very different impression from those taken at points P, Q, R, and S, yet they belong to the same profile.

Guidelines for adjusting treatment

- Changes in insulin dose should be made only once or twice weekly except in times of illness when more frequent changes may be needed, or in those following dose adjustment for normal eating (DAFNE) (see page 29).
- Changes in insulin dose at any one time should normally be kept within 10% of the existing daily dose—for example, a change of four units may be made in a patient taking a total daily dose of 40 units.

The following issues need consideration:

- type of insulin (considered in detail on page 19)
- frequency of administration of insulin
- dose of insulin in units
- carbohydrate distribution.

The patterns of the blood glucose profile need to be understood and are much more important than single, randomly taken readings. When consistent daily fluctuations of blood glucose have been shown, treatment should be modified, aiming chiefly to eliminate hypoglycaemic episodes, and thereafter to obtain better control by increasing the blood glucose in the troughs and decreasing it at the peaks. There are several ways of achieving fine glucose control.

Self assessment of diabetic control in Type 2 diabetes

Home blood glucose monitoring is of value for many (though not necessarily all) patients with Type 2 diabetes, as it is for those with Type 1 diabetes. Those taking oral hypoglycaemic agents or on diet alone have the option to monitor their control by either self blood glucose measurement or regular urine testing. Measurement of the fasting blood glucose two or three times weekly in those on diet alone provides a valuable guide to control, while the addition of some postprandial readings in those taking oral hypoglycaemic agents also provides important information.

Continuous subcutaneous insulin infusion (CSSI)

CSSI was introduced 25 years ago by workers at Guy's Hospital in London, and now the development of more reliable and more sophisticated pumps brings distinct advantages in specific indications to approximately 2 to 5% of those with Type 1 diabetes. A small improvement in overall diabetic control compared with optimised injection regimens can be achieved without necessarily aggravating or indeed actually reducing problems from hypoglycaemia. CSSI is not suitable for those with psychological or psychiatric problems.

Hazards

Experience has virtually eliminated earlier hazards of excessive problems from hypoglycaemia or, because of the very small insulin depot, higher rates of diabetic ketoacidosis. All patients should have a supply of insulin pens or syringes in case of pump failure.

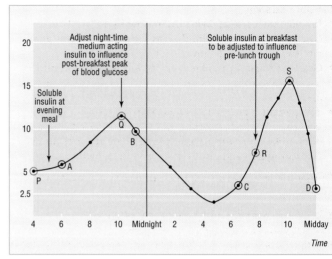

Adjustments after assessment of blood glucose profiles. Note the apparent different shape of the profile if readings are taken at points ABCD or PQRS

To increase blood glucose in the troughs

- Eat more carbohydrate at or before the times when blood glucose values are at their lowest, usually mid-morning and at bedtime; the exact amount of extra carbohydrate can be determined only by trial and error
- Reduce the dose of insulin before the trough
- Premeal hypoglycaemia can be ameliorated by substituting short acting insulin with a very short acting insulin analogue

To decrease blood glucose in the peaks

- Reduce by a little the amount of carbohydrate taken at the meals which precede the peaks by two or three hours
- Increase the dose of insulin before the peak

Soluble insulin should be altered to change blood glucose concentrations during the following six hours. Medium acting insulin should be altered to change blood glucose during the following six to 12 hours. The duration of insulin action varies considerably however in individual patients

To decrease fasting hyperglycaemia

- Increase predinner medium (or long) acting insulin.
- If that provokes night-time hypoglycaemia, then split the predinner insulin into two parts, retaining the short acting insulin before dinner and taking medium acting insulin at bedtime; or consider changing the medium acting insulin component to insulin glargine

To lessen nocturnal hypoglycaemia

- Reduce the evening medium acting insulin dose
- Check that the patient is taking their bedtime snack
- Check bedtime blood glucose, taking additional carbohydrate if it is less than 5·0 to 6·0 mmol/l
- Split predinner insulin dose, or consider changing to insulin glargine

For a detailed description of the use of individual insulin types, see chapters 6 and 8

Infusion strategy
- Initially reduce total daily insulin dose by 30%.
- Give half the daily insulin dose as the constant basal pump rate (usually around 1 unit/hour).
- Give half the daily insulin dose divided between the three main meals, giving the insulin boost immediately before the meal.
- The patient is taught to count carbohydrate portions (see page 12) and thereafter will give the bolus doses in direct relation to the amount of carbohydrate consumed (for example, 1 unit for every 10 g of carbohydrate).

During the first few days adjustments need to be made as follows:

- basal rate determined by assessment of fasting and 3 am blood glucose readings
- preprandial boosts are adjusted by assessment of postprandial blood glucose readings.

  Note: Specific instructions are given for exercise, and basal rates should be reduced during and after exercise.

Indications for CSSI
- Management of patients with frequent unpredictable hypoglycaemic episodes
- For control of the dawn hyperglycaemic phenomenon when conventional, optimised regimens have failed
- For greater flexibility of lifestyle
- In pregnancy when conventional methods fail
- For patients employed on shift rotas who are not able to achieve glycaemic control on multiple injections

Optimal results are achieved using non-associating, monomeric insulin analogues, for example, lispro insulin (Humalog), or Insulin Aspart (Novo Rapid)

Training of patients is undertaken by the nurse educators and a 24-hour duty scheme is needed to deal with emergencies

Dose adjustment for normal eating (DAFNE)

A more liberal dietary pattern for Type 1 diabetic patients has become possible by using the DAFNE approach, ideal for some people who thus regain considerable freedom while at the same time maintaining good control. It is based on:

- a 5-day structured, group education programme delivered by quality assured diabetes educators
- the educational approach is based on adult educational principles to facilitate new learning
- two injections of medium acting insulin each day (see page 21)
- injections of short acting insulin every time meals are taken
- testing blood glucose before each injection.

  This programme enables people to eat more or less what they like when they like, and not to eat if they do not wish to do so. It depends on a quantitative understanding of the carbohydrate values of individual foods, and calculating by trial and error the correct amount of soluble insulin needed for a specified quantity of carbohydrate, developing an insulin/carbohydrate ratio for each individual patient.

  DAFNE has been used in continental Europe for many years: the approach is popular and gives considerable benefits to some patients. Good diabetic control can be achieved without any increase in hypoglycaemia and at the same time there is improvement in the quality of life.

The photographs of blood glucose meters and the finger pricking devices are reproduced with permission from MediSense and Roche Diagnostics.

The story of Mrs B-J continues: attending the clinic

Then I began my regular visits to the clinic, which I think was every three weeks at first. This was held upstairs in the pathology laboratory, with the doctors in a small room off. I was fascinated by all that was going on there; so many bottles, test tubes, Bunsen burners, etc., as the tests were done there for all the hospital. The waiting room was very small and if a dozen patients attended it was a crowd, for there were only about 200 diabetic patients on the hospital's roll.

  I remember Dr RD Lawrence vividly. He always looked very smart in black jacket and striped trousers and a black bow. He took a great interest in the children, and I felt encouraged that such a great man was also diabetic.

  Over the years the number of patients attending the clinic increased. We often had long waits and were obliged to listen to very gruesome tales from some of the adults. Shortly afterwards, the children's clinic was arranged, and I attended with quite a few others on Saturday mornings.

  There were "elevenses" laid on, and an ice cream could be had as a portion. At first, ice cream was not considered suitable for diabetics even as part of the diet, so I was happy to find this was no longer so, and a Walls twopenny brick was a real treat.

7 The unstable Type 1 diabetic patient

Blood glucose concentrations inevitably oscillate considerably over 24 hours in many Type 1 diabetic patients. If these swings are used as a definition of instability then such patients might be classified as unstable. Indeed the ardent desire of some doctors to "stabilise" these patients sometimes leads the patient to undertake innumerable blood tests, to keep obsessional records, and to make themselves thoroughly miserable. The failure to succeed leads to recriminations, admissions to hospital, and absence from work. This form of physician-induced, unstable diabetes is made worse by the inappropriate use of home blood glucose monitoring. It needs considerable patience to unravel the effects of such advice, but a more relaxed approach, together with fewer tests, can have a remarkably beneficial effect.

Very unstable diabetes (sometimes described as "brittle") disrupts the lives of a small group of insulin treated diabetic patients, with repeated admissions to hospital due either to hypoglycaemia or ketoacidosis. Homelife, school, and work are totally disrupted. With very few exceptions, this is probably not a special type of diabetes; it most commonly occurs in teenage girls, it is almost always temporary, and problems appear to vanish as life itself stabilises with employment or marriage.

Management of disruptive diabetes demands time and patience; the doctor must identify any technical errors, recommend the best possible diabetic treatment, search for intercurrent illness, and seek social or psychological problems which might cause the patient to manipulate his or her diabetes. Some elderly patients also experience serious problems from violent swings of blood glucose. Loss of support at home following separation or bereavement can be added to the specific problems already described.

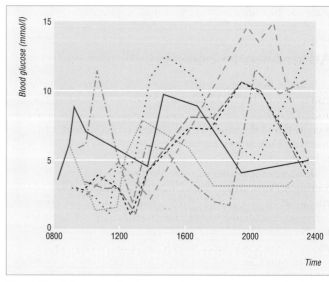

Chaotic blood glucose profiles in one patient over seven consecutive days

Disruptive diabetes has several causes, ranging from simple technical errors to gross deceptions of great ingenuity

Solving technical problems

After all the technical issues have been checked, the dose and type of insulin should be adjusted to the best possible regimen (ideal insulin regimens have been described elsewhere). Some obsessional patients respond well to a reduction of the number of daily injections. A few unstable diabetic patients may benefit from continuous subcutaneous insulin infusion, which may also alleviate unpleasant hypoglycaemic episodes.

If recurrent hypoglycaemic episodes are the chief problem then careful education is needed to eliminate them (see chapter 8); careful attention needs to be given not only to the dose of insulin but also to the timing and amount of food, the effects of exercise, and the judicious use of home measurement of blood glucose. Sometimes excessive amounts of insulin, especially soluble insulin, may cause severe hypoglycaemia. Improvement results either from reducing the dose or changing the insulin regimen.

In a few women menstruation regularly causes severe upset of diabetes; control usually deteriorates in the premenstrual phase, causing ketoacidosis at times, followed by an increase in insulin requirement and sometimes troublesome hypoglycaemia. A carefully planned campaign of insulin adjustment usually overcomes this problem.

Identifying technical problems
- The technique of injecting insulin should be meticulously checked
- Injection sites should be inspected
- Equipment needs to be scrutinised
- Sometimes, especially in elderly patients, reduced visual acuity makes measurement of the insulin dose extremely inaccurate
- The brand of insulin itself should be checked
- Techniques of blood glucose testing must be observed and checked with laboratory results
- Adequate understanding of diet should be verified

Above all, patients need encouragement and restoration of self-confidence together with the reassurance that they are neither physically nor mentally abnormal. The telephone number of the doctor or nurse offers added security. If at all possible unstable patients should not be admitted to hospital. If all these measures fail, however, and life is still disrupted by diabetes, then an admission is after all required.

Admission to hospital

In hospital the nursing staff take over the administration of insulin completely—both the procedure of drawing up the insulin and giving the injections. If some measure of stability is then achieved the patient's equipment is returned for self injection: if chaos resumes it seems likely that the patient is either incompetent or cheating.

If diabetes continues to cause disruption even when the nursing staff are giving insulin injections, some form of manipulation should be suspected. Some patients use great ingenuity; insulin may just be concealed in a locker, but it has also been found inside transistor radios, in the false bottoms of jewellery boxes, and taped outside hospital lavatory windows.

Manipulation should be suspected in patients whose lives are totally disrupted by their diabetes. A careful history may reveal slips which give the vital clue. For instance, one teenager developed profound hypoglycaemia two days after apparently "stopping insulin"; another, whose life was spent in and out of hospital with hypoglycaemia or ketoacidosis, claimed to be perfectly stable in-between, presenting a whole volume of negative urine tests. Even constant insulin infusion does not necessarily solve the problem, especially when the patient replaces the insulin in the syringe with water. When there is strong evidence of manipulation, try hinting at the possibility to the patient or their parents but without accusation. The technique is sometimes successful and gratitude considerable.

Emotional, social, or psychiatric causes underlie disruptive diabetes and the desire to manipulate the situation to cause widespread havoc among families. Teenage defiance is a common cause. Quiet support of families at these difficult times helps to overcome what is almost always a temporary phase. Careful enquiry should establish whether there is family strife, and family counselling is often valuable. Psychiatric advice should only be sought if there is evidence of a psychiatric disorder. It is a huge advantage to work closely with a sympathetic liaison psychiatrist who understands the specific problems of diabetes and is unthreatening to patients; otherwise, confrontation with a psychiatrist may provoke even more aggression. Nonetheless, a few patients remain incapable of independent existence, and then community care strategies are essential.

Various disorders, especially infections and some endocrine disorders, may alter the insulin requirements, although they rarely cause the type of instability already described.

> At one clinic of yours which I attended, you asked me if I was taking overdoses. I was stupid and did not admit this until December 1981. I am still not as well balanced as I would like, but I am better than I was.

Letter from a patient

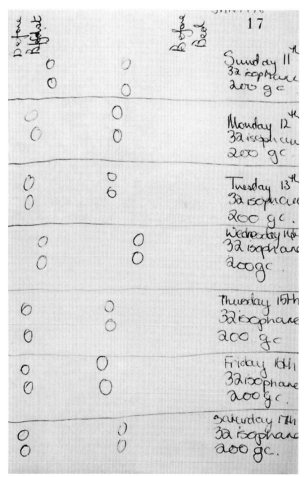

Falsified urine chart from a very unstable teenage patient

8 Hypoglycaemia

Hypoglycaemia is the major hazard of insulin treatment, and problems have increased in the drive to achieve "tight control". Patients may experience the symptoms of hypoglycaemia when the blood concentration is less than $3.0 \, \text{mmol/l}$. However, individual susceptibility varies considerably and it is interesting that some patients whose control has been persistently very poor for long periods appear to experience hypoglycaemic symptoms at levels a little above this. The risks of hazard from hypoglycaemia are small in most patients, but because they exist at all, patients taking insulin are barred from certain occupations such as driving trains or buses. All patients taking insulin whose diabetes is reasonably well controlled will experience hypoglycaemia at some stage. At its mildest, it is no more than a slight inconvenience, but at its severest, when unconsciousness can occur, it is both a hazard and an embarrassment. Furthermore, manipulative patients can use hypoglycaemia to threaten family and friends. This sword of Damocles is ever present once insulin treatment has started, and the need to use measures to avoid it requires constant, indeed lifelong, vigilance. Hypoglycaemia occurs infrequently in patients taking oral hypoglycaemics.

Hypoglycaemia ("hypo" "insulin reaction")

This is when the blood sugar goes too low in diabetics taking insulin

Symptoms are sweating, shaking, tingling round the mouth, hazy eyesight or seeing double, slow thinking, in children naughtiness

Causes are late meal, too little carbohydrate, extra exercise, too much insulin.

Cure is to take carboydrate—preferably three dextrosol tablets, glucose, sugar (two large lumps), barley sugar, Lucozade followed by a small snack

Symptoms will soon wear off

If in doubt about an attack, take sugar

Always carry some form of SUGAR with you

Symptoms

Most patients experience the early warning symptoms of hypoglycaemia and can take sugar before more serious symptoms develop. These warning symptoms are well known and are described in the box. Tremulousness and sweating are by far the commonest symptoms, while circumoral paraesthesiae is the most specific. Many patients have highly individual symptoms of hypoglycaemia which range from quite inexplicable sensations to peripheral paraesthesiae.

In three patients carpal tunnel compression resulted in tingling fingers when they were hypoglycaemic, representing their sole warning. Neuroglyopenic symptoms and diminished cognitive function follow if corrective action is not taken, with progressive confusion and eventually unconsciousness and occasionally convulsions. There is a prolonged debate as to whether recurrent hypoglycaemia causes long-term intellectual decline; the evidence in general is unconvincing although major and recurrent episodes in childhood may have an adverse effect in this regard.

Patients who become unconscious from hypoglycaemia need urgent treatment. Brain damage and death do not normally occur because the blood glucose concentration tends to increase spontaneously as the effect of the insulin wears off and the normal counter-regulatory responses become effective. Many diabetics, especially children, need reassurance that they will not die in their sleep. Nevertheless, a very small number of otherwise unexplained deaths at night have been reported in Type 1 diabetic patients (described as the "dead in bed" syndrome) and no precise cause has ever been established. Deaths from prolonged hypoglycaemia are most likely to occur after insulin overdoses, as a result either of a suicide or murder attempt, but even in these circumstances most patients recover.

Symptoms of hypoglycaemia

• **Early warning**	Shaking, trembling
	Sweating
	Pins and needles in lips and tongue
	Hunger
	Palpitations
	Headache (occasionally)
Neuroglycopenia	
• **Mild**	Double vision
	Difficulty in concentrating
	Slurring of speech
• **More advanced**	Confusion
	Change of behaviour
	Truculence
	Naughtiness in children
• **Unconsciousness**	Restlessness with sweating
	Epileptic fits, especially in children
	Hemiplegia, especially in older people (but rare)

Observation of a hypoglycaemic attack

"When she is having a hypo she gives the impression of being drunk. The change in her behaviour is sudden and very noticeable. She slurs her words and appears drowsy. There is lots and lots of yawning. If she is still in the state of which she can walk, she will bump in to things and knock things over and be generally clumsy. She will hardly be aware of where she is or who she is talking to. She rambles"

Diminished awareness of hypoglycaemia

This is the problem which all insulin treated patients dread, and at some stage it affects up to one quarter of Type 1 diabetic patients. It occurs when patients do not experience the early warning symptoms and directly develop diminished cognitive function which prevents them from taking the required preventive action. In this situation, help is required from a third party. This commonly occurs in the home when friends and relations observe the person to be slow-witted with a vacant expression and perspiring face. They may be taciturn, truculent or even obstructive, sometimes refusing to take sugar when advised, although many learn to accept this advice. This state of cognitive impairment can persist for some considerable time, long enough for abnormal behaviour to be noticed during driving, even for several miles; shoppers in the High Street may be unaware that they are shoplifting. If corrective action is not taken, the more serious state of unconsciousness already described can occur.

Night-time hypoglycaemia is very common, usually occurring between 3 and 6 am. The blood glucose concentration often falls below the hypoglycaemic threshold; levels as low as 1·0 mmol/l are not rare, and are known to cause electroencephalogram abnormalities even in the absence of symptoms. Many people become very restless when hypoglycaemic; this is recognised most frequently by the spouse who takes the necessary remedial action. Profound sweating is common, sometimes necessitating a change of nightclothes or bedclothes and may be the only manifestation that hypoglycaemia has occurred. Convulsions are not rare, and some patients wake in the morning with a bitten tongue as the only indication that this may have occured.

Recurrent hypoglycaemia is the principal underlying cause leading to diminished awareness of hypoglycaemia, with dangerous impairment of cognitive function its chief manifestation. It is therefore most likely to occur in those who are most tightly controlled, and was manifest in the famous Diabetes Control and Complications Trial (DCCT) in which severe hypoglycaemia occurred three times more often in the tightly controlled group of patients. This cause outweighs all others, although the use of β adrenergic blockers has the same effect in a small number of patients. Autonomic neuropathy is not normally the cause of diminished warning, and the contentious role of human insulin in this regard has led some patients to change back to animal insulins, though scientific evidence of harm is still lacking. Diminished warning also increases with lengthening duration of diabetes.

Why does recurrent hypoglycaemia beget loss of warning? The answer probably lies in the readjustment of the threshold of sensitivity of a glucose sensor in the hypothalamic region of the central nervous system. This alters the hierarchy of responses to hypoglycaemia. Thus, the hypoglycaemic symptoms and counter regulatory responses, instead of occurring at a blood glucose just above 3·0 mmol/l, develop at a lower level, rather less than 2·0 mmol/l. Because in either case the loss of cognitive function occurs around 2·8 mmol/l it is clear that, in cases of diminished hypoglycaemic awareness reduced cognitive function develops before hypoglycaemic warning symptoms.

Recent research has also shown that by eliminating recurrent hypoglycaemia it is possible to restore the normal sequence of events when blood glucose falls, thus also restoring adequate warning. It is therefore necessary to eliminate as far as possible all hypoglycaemic episodes, even those occurring

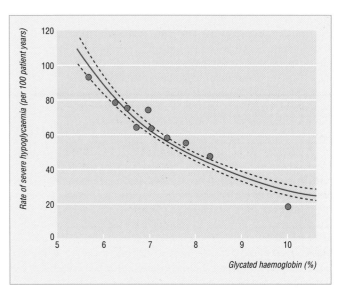

Relationship between glycated haemoglobin and hypoglycaemia rates shown in the DCCT study

Avoiding hypoglycaemia can restore proper warning symptoms. Patients should try to avoid blood glucose levels < 4·0 mmol.

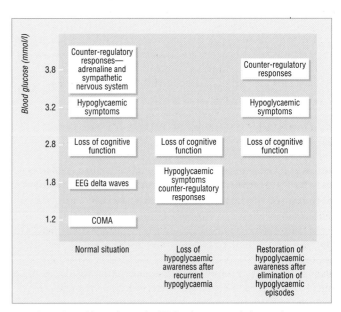

Loss of warning of hypoglycaemia (EEG=electroencephalogram)

quietly at night. This can often be achieved simply by reducing the insulin dose, ensuring adequate carbohydrate intake and to some extent relaxing overall diabetic control in the interest of safety. It is much more difficult, yet possible, to eliminate hypoglycaemia and retain optimal control of diabetes. The acquired skill of the diabetes team and the co-operation of patients is needed if this is to be done, and the time and resources needed are considerable. The introduction of programmes such as blood glucose awareness training (BGAT), in which patients are taught how to recognise the most subtle symptoms of early hypoglycaemia, can be very effective in reducing serious hypoglycaemia and thus helping to restore adequate warning.

A questionnaire which helps physicians to assess whether a patient has diminished awareness of hypoglycaemia is shown in Appendix 1.

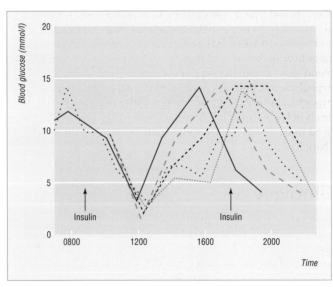

Reproducible blood glucose profiles in one patient during five consecutive days, showing the times of blood glucose "troughs" when hypoglycaemia is most likely to occur

Causes of hypoglycaemia

In every patient taking insulin the blood glucose concentration shows peaks and troughs, which can be most clearly shown by home measurements of blood glucose. Since the lowest blood glucose concentrations occur at different times in each patient, it is a great advantage if individual patients know when their own troughs are likely to occur. The commonest times are before lunch and during the night. Some patients in their constant fear of developing diabetic complications drive their blood glucose levels ever lower with disastrous consequences in terms of hypoglycaemia.

Severe physical activity, such as swimming very long distances, is a powerful stimulus of hypoglycaemia, and as much as 40 to 50 g additional carbohydrate may be needed to prevent it. Hypoglycaemia in these situations is sometimes delayed for several hours. Several well-known sportsmen and women with diabetes show considerable ingenuity and perseverance in the way in which they cope with their diabetes during international competitions, by individual attention to food and insulin intake, carefully timed blood glucose monitoring, and ready availability of sugary fluids such as Lucozade at exactly the right moment.

Hypoglycaemia is particularly likely to occur shortly after stabilisation of new patients, as their insulin requirements may decline considerably; their insulin dose should therefore always be reduced before they leave hospital.

Hypoglycaemia is also troublesome when insulin requirements insidiously decrease during the evolution of such conditions as Addison's disease, hypopituitarism, and malabsorption syndromes.

Events likely to provoke hypoglycaemic attacks
- Insufficient carbohydrate in meals
- Delayed meals
- Increased physical activity
- Errors of insulin dosage
- Erratic insulin absorption from areas of fat hypertrophy at injection sites

Treatment and prevention of hypoglycaemia

Much of the skill required to manage insulin treated diabetic patients is therefore devoted to achieving adequate control of diabetes, yet avoiding hypoglycaemia. There are quite straightforward measures which many patients neglect: they must therefore at all times carry a supply of glucose both on their person and in their cars, and take 10 to 20 g at the first warning symptoms, preferably followed by a carbohydrate snack. The late RD Lawrence always demanded that his patients should demonstrate that they were carrying their sugar supply with them. This can take the form of sugar lumps, sweets (non-diabetic), sugar gel or dextrose tablets.

Items containing 10 g of carbohydrate
• Milk	200 ml (⅓ pint)
• Lucozade	60 ml (4 tablespoons)
• Ribena	15 ml (1 tablespoon)
• Coca Cola	90 ml
• Sugar	2 teaspoons
• Sugar lumps (small)	3
• Dextrosol tablets	3

They should take ample carbohydrate at times when blood glucose troughs occur, notably mid-morning and bedtime, and they must take appropriate amounts of additional carbohydrate before and during vigorous exercise. Careful blood glucose monitoring plays a crucial part in avoiding hypoglycaemic episodes, and helps to restore warning of hypoglycaemia. Patients should try to avoid blood glucose levels below 4·0 mmol/l. Appropriate insulin regimens that need to be devised for individual patients are described in chapters 5 and 6.

Glucagon

Glucagon is a hormone produced by the A-cells of the pancreatic islets. It raises the blood glucose by mobilising the glycogen stores in the liver (and therefore will not work after prolonged starvation). It is given in a 1 mg dose by injection most conveniently intramuscularly. It can also be used subcutaneously or intravenously and is effective in five to 10 minutes. It is of great value for bystanders of severely hypoglycaemic patients who are unable to take oral glucose, and can be injected by family members, nurses or doctors. It is valuable in relieving stress in a home where a diabetic patient, often a child, is prone to recurrent disabling attacks of hypoglycaemia.

Unconsciousness

In cases where the patient has lapsed into severe unconsciousness, treatment in hospital is urgently needed. The unconscious patient should be placed in the recovery position, and the airway maintained. Blood should be taken for blood glucose analysis and the sample should be kept in case the patient fails to respond to treatment since the possibility always exists that the coma has another cause. Intravenous glucose is given using 50 ml of 20% glucose solution. The more concentrated 50% solution is highly irritant and should no longer be used. The response is usually immediate but if not, a further dose should be given after five to 10 minutes followed by an infusion of 10% glucose. Once consciousness is restored and a history can be taken, the patient should be fed with longer acting carbohydrate to prevent recurrence. If recovery does not occur rapidly, blood glucose measurement should be repeated and another cause for the coma must be sought. If hypoglycaemia has been profound, cerebral oedema can occur and may require treatment with dexamethasone or mannitol. After recovery appropriate adjustment must be made to the diabetic treatment in order to avoid further episodes, and the patient should be carefully reviewed in the diabetic clinic.

Hypoglycaemia due to oral hypoglycaemics

This may occur during treatment with sulphonylureas and similar agents (but not with metformin) especially in some confused elderly patients who either inadvertently take additional tablets or omit their meals. It is treated in the same way as described above. These patients usually require admission to hospital for continuous glucose infusion to avoid relapse into hypoglycaemia, which often occurs until the drug has been cleared from the circulation.

Dr Charles Fletcher's account of hypoglycaemia

My main problem has always been hypoglycaemia. At first I was nearly always aware of it by day and woke at night, because of the adrenaline response. But, particularly in the past 20 years, it gradually became more difficult. I may now feel normal and do ordinary tasks quite easily with blood sugar as low as 2·5 mmol/l (45 mg/100 ml). Sometimes diplopia, dysphasia, weariness, or inability to think may lead me to do a blood sugar. But I often become too muddled to know what is wrong, and I have had to thank my wife, my children, and many generations of housemen, registrars, and secretaries for spotting these low levels on many occasions. Before I retired 50% glucose was always available with syringe in a drawer in my desk. I became quite used to a quiet registrar's voice in outpatients (and elsewhere) saying, "I think, sir, a little extravenous glucose might help". Lucozade has been invaluable. I always have it available in the car, in the office, and at home. It is acceptably free from sugariness, it saves me chewing and choking on dry glucose tablets, and it is rapidly absorbed. My wife finds it much easier to get me to drink this than to take any other form of sugar when I am severely hypoglycaemic and refuse to acknowledge it. I have made it a rule, which I now keep, even when semi-comatose, that if my wife—or anyone else—tells me to take sugar I do so however sure I may be that I'm not hypoglycaemic. They have only been wrong on rare occasions. I am very sensitive to exercise, but for some reason I find it difficult always to suck prophylactic sweets on country walks or when digging or mowing in the garden.

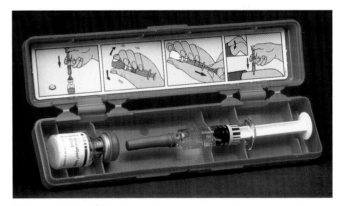

Glucagon injection kit

Conclusions

Any serious hypoglycaemic episodes can to some extent be regarded as a failure of the doctor, the patient or the treatment regimen itself. It should provoke a serious inquiry to establish the cause and to discover if it is likely to recur. The opportunity for the necessary education should be taken, and patients should be encouraged to carry a diabetic identification card. Finally, the professional attending the patient, whether doctor or nurse, has a duty to inform people who have had an episode of severe hypoglycaemia comprising diminished cognitive function resulting from diminished awareness of hypoglycaemia to stop driving and inform the Driver and Vehicle Licensing Agency. They should also avoid any other potentially dangerous activity. The endeavour to avoid hypoglycaemia needs to be maintained, and patients need considerable support to this end at almost every diabetic consultation throughout life.

The figure showing the relationship between glycated haemoglobin and hypoglycaemia rates is adapted from Donnelly R, et al *BMJ* 2000;320:1062-6. The photograph of the glucacon injection kit is with permission from Novo Nordisk. Dr Charles Fletcher's account of hypoglycaemia is from *BMJ* 1980;280:1115-16.

The story of Mrs B-J continued: hypoglycaemia

When I was 12 I was sent to The Old Palace School in Croydon. Never having done any gymnastics, I was surprised at what was expected of me at the new school. Rope climbing, parallel bars, and marching up and down the long hall where kings had been entertained by archbishops, I was soon very hypo and staggering about like a drunk. This disrupted the session so much that finally I was banned from gym and all other sports. My fellow diabetic, Barbara, had also been banned, but it did not worry me too much. But it was a bitter blow when I was told I would not be allowed to take part in the school pageant "in case I was ill"! My mother went up to see Sister and assured her I would have plenty of sugar etc., but to no avail. Gentle nuns can be very obstinate and quite hardhearted at times.

9 Diabetic ketoacidosis and management of diabetes during surgery

Ketoacidosis

Ketoacidosis results from a lack of insulin. In practice it is usually due to:

- stopping insulin or reducing the dose either in error or deliberately
- resistance to insulin during infections or other intercurrent illness
- the unrecognised onset of Type 1 diabetes.

The clinical onset of ketoacidosis occurs over hours or days. Symptoms of uncontrolled diabetes are always present. Vomiting in Type 1 diabetic patients is always serious. Patients usually consult their doctors during the preceding days, but the presence of uncontrolled diabetes is frequently overlooked. Diabetic control should always be assessed if a diabetic patient becomes unwell for any reason. Many cases of ketoacidosis could be prevented.

Preventing ketoacidosis: sick day rules
During any illness or infection the blood glucose concentration tends to increase and diabetic control deteriorates. Most patients then need a larger dose of insulin than usual, and some who normally take tablets may need insulin just during the illness. The increased need for insulin occurs even when the appetite declines or vomiting begins.

Every insulin treated patient should understand that insulin should never be stopped. Stopping or even reducing insulin during the course of an illness often leads to diabetic ketoacidosis.

When a diabetic person is ill the normal insulin dose should be continued, carbohydrate taken in some palatable fluid form, and the blood tested regularly—four times a day if necessary. If blood glucose readings greater than 15 mmol/l are obtained the dose of insulin should be increased. Additional doses of insulin (about 8 units) may also be given at noon or bedtime when control is very poor. It is preferable to make these adjustments with short acting (soluble) insulin if this is available. If vomiting continues without remission for more than a few hours, admission to hospital for treatment with intravenous fluids and insulin is advisable to prevent ketoacidosis.

Assessment of blood or urine ketones during illness is helpful. Using the new blood ketone meters, readings of 1·0-3·0 mmol/l taken in conjunction with the blood glucose reading usually indicate the need for additional insulin; readings should be repeated within two to four hours. If they persist or increase above 3·0 mmol/l, specialist advice is required from the hospital clinic staff. Ketonuria can be detected using Ketostix, which are readily available.

Recognising ketoacidosis
Dehydration is the most obvious clinical feature of patients with ketoacidosis. They are also drowsy, but rarely unconscious— "diabetic coma" is an inappropriate description; they are often overbreathing, but not usually breathless; their breath smells of acetone (though many people cannot smell this); and many also have the gastric splash. In more severe cases patients are

<table>
<tr><th colspan="2">Causes of diabetic ketoacidosis</th></tr>
<tr><td>• Omission or reduction of insulin dose</td><td>27%</td></tr>
<tr><td>• Previously unknown diabetes</td><td>22%</td></tr>
<tr><td>• Infection</td><td>17%</td></tr>
<tr><td>• Miscellaneous</td><td>16%</td></tr>
<tr><td>• No cause found</td><td>18%</td></tr>
</table>

King's College Hospital 1968

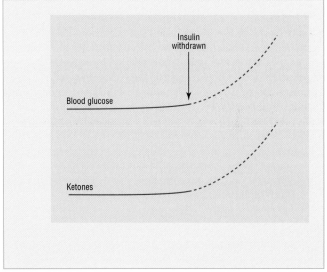

Ketoacidosis

Prevention of ketoacidosis
Insulin should never be stopped

Insulin dose during illness or infection
During illness or infection your blood glucose level may rise, causing you to feel dry, thirsty and pass too much urine. The blood glucose is also likely to increase

You MUST continue to take your normal insulin dose NEVER stop it. You may need an increased dose if your blood tests are bad. If you are vomiting, consult your doctor or the diabetic clinic at once. If you are unable to eat, take your carbohydrate portions in liquid form—for example, milk, Lucozade, Ribena

Test your blood twice a day or even more frequently

If you continue to feel unwell, consult your doctor.

Features of ketoacidosis
- Drowsiness
- Dehydration
- Overbreathing
- Acetone on breath
- Hypotension
- Gastric splash

hypothermic (even in the presence of infection) and hypotensive. Hyperosmolar non-ketotic (HONK) patients are usually grossly dehydrated but without overbreathing or the smell of acetone. Inexperienced clinicians often have difficulty in recognising patients with this condition, especially when they seem deceptively well.

Diagnosis
The diagnosis of ketoacidosis is confirmed by laboratory tests.

- **Blood glucose** concentrations may range from slightly increased to extreme hyperglycaemia. The blood glucose concentration itself does not usually indicate the severity of the illness, although most patients are seriously unwell when it is greater than 30 mmol/l.
- **Blood acid-base status** pH ranges from 6·9 to normal. The bicarbonate level is depressed.
- **Plasma ketones** are easily detectable with a ketone meter and exceed 3·0 mmol/l.
- **Urine test** shows heavy glycosuria and ketonuria.
- **Electrolytes**: the serum potassium concentration is either normal or raised, and very rarely low. This measurement is vital, and life-saving treatment is needed to maintain potassium values in the normal range. The sodium concentration is normal or reduced, and urea and creatinine concentrations are often raised through dehydration.
- **Blood count**: if a blood count is performed the white cell count is often spuriously raised to 15-20 × 10⁹/l even in the absence of infection.

    Serum amylase is sometimes moderately elevated in patients with diabetic ketoacidosis: it is of salivary origin and need not be indicative of pancreatitis

Treatment
Patients should be treated in an area where there they can be observed regularly, preferably by staff familiar with managing this condition, in a high dependency area, or if very ill in intensive care.

- Insert a nasogastric tube if consciousness is impaired. Do not allow any fluids by mouth; if patients are thirsty they may suck ice.
- Give intravenous fluids. The regimen needs to be modified according to age, weight, and the presence of cardiac disease. In seriously ill patients and all those with cardiac disease a catheter for measuring central venous pressure is essential. A suitable regimen for most patients is shown in the box; 0·9% saline is used.
- The fluid should be changed to 10% dextrose once the blood glucose concentration has fallen to less than 10 mmol/l. The rate of infusion is determined by individual need but at this stage should probably be about one litre every eight hours.
- Start intravenous soluble insulin immediately. If there is any delay in obtaining intravenous access. Soluble insulin (20 units) can be given immediately intramuscularly.

Insulin treatment
Intravenous insulin: soluble insulin is diluted in 0·9% saline in a syringe, at the concentration of 1 unit/ml. It is given by infusion pump at 6 units/h (0·1 units/kg/h for children) until the blood glucose concentration is less than 10 mmol/l. Blood glucose should fall at a rate of about 5·0 mmol/l/h, and plasma ketones should fall at the same time. When the blood glucose is less than 10 mmol/l, the dose may be reduced to 3 units/h. Higher infusion rates are rarely needed; when they are needed

Tests for ketoacidosis
- Blood glucose
- Serum potassium and sodium
- Acid-base status
- Urea, creatinine
- Plasma or urine ketones
- Blood count
- Blood culture (when indicated)

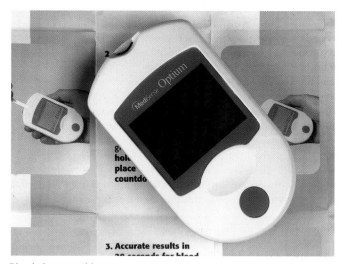

Blood glucose and ketone meter

Treatment of ketoacidosis

Physiological saline:*	1 l in first half hour	-½ h
	1 l over next hour	½-1½ h
	1 l over next hour	1½-2½ h
	1 l over next 2 hours	2½-4½ h
	1 l over next 3 hours	4½-7½ h
	1 l over next 4 hours	7½-11½ h
Total:	6 l	11½ h

*Change to 10% dextrose when blood glucose is less than 10 mmol/l in insulin resistant patients the rate should be doubled or quadrupled, etc. If the patient is not responding, medical staff should check the equipment for pump failure, blockage or leakage. The insulin infusion is continued until the patient is well enough to eat. The changeover to subcutaneous insulin should be made before breakfast. Preprandial subcutaneous soluble insulin is then given and intravenous insulin discontinued after the meal. Intravenous insulin should not be stopped before subcutaneous insulin has been given (see below).

Intramuscular insulin is used only when an infusion pump is not available. Soluble insulin 20 units is given as a loading dose, than 6 units every hour until blood glucose is less than 10 mmol/l, then continued at two hourly intervals. As with intravenous insulin, higher doses are rarely needed.

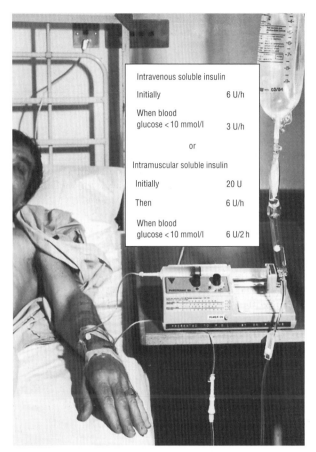

Intravenous soluble insulin	
Initially	6 U/h
When blood glucose < 10 mmol/l	3 U/h
or	
Intramuscular soluble insulin	
Initially	20 U
Then	6 U/h
When blood glucose < 10 mmol/l	6 U/2 h

Giving intravenous insulin

Potassium and sodium bicarbonate

Potassium chloride administration should usually start at about the second hour, preferably not before the serum potassium concentration is known. It should be withheld in exceptional cases of oliguria or anuria, or if the serum potassium value remains above 5·0 mmol/l. After the second hour, or earlier if the initial serum potassium value is normal or less than 4·0 mmol/l, 20 mmol potassium chloride should be added to each litre of saline. If the serum potassium value falls below 3·5 mmol/l, 40 mmol should be used in each litre. The exact amount should be determined by serial serum potassium measurements—every two hours at first, then every four hours—and serum potassium maintained between 4·0 and 5·0 mmol/l. An electrocardiographic monitor should be set up; however, there is no substitute for serial potassium measurements.

Sodium bicarbonate is not normally beneficial and is not given unless the blood pH value is less than 7·0 or the patient is shocked. If it is needed, aliquots of sodium bicarbonate (500 ml of 1·26%) with added potassium chloride (15 mmol) should be given. This can be repeated if there is no response within one hour and if the patient's condition remains serious.
Note: Never use sodium bicarbonate 8·4% concentration.

Treatment of the underlying condition

Underlying disease should be sought, especially respiratory or urinary infections, which may not be obvious at the onset. Blood culture, culture of the midstream specimen of urine, and chest radiography are performed. There is no need to give antibiotics routinely. Abdominal pain may occur, especially in young patients with severe ketoacidosis. It is vital to discover whether there is indeed an intra-abdominal cause needing attention if the pain does not resolve rapidly.

HONK patients

Blood glucose in these patients can be extremely high without ketosis or acidosis. Management is the same as that for ketoacidosis, except that 0·45% saline is given if the serum sodium value is greater than 150 mmol/l, and a lower rate of insulin infusion (3 units/h) is often sufficient. In shocked and dehydrated patients prophylactic, low dose, subcutaneous heparin is considered.

Lactic acidosis

These patients are profoundly ill and the cause of the acidosis must be sought and rigorously treated. They are often very insulin resistant due to serious intercurrent illness, and need large amounts of sodium bicarbonate. Absence of a raised plasma ketone level excludes ketoacidosis as the cause of the metabolic acidosis. Metformin induced lactic acidosis should be borne in mind.

Potassium chloride administration

Serum value (mmol/l)	< 3·5	3·5-4·0	4·0-5·0	> 5·0
Administer	40 mmol/l	30 mmol/l	20 mmol/l	0

Patients who develop HONK are often elderly or West Indian, and they often turn out to have Type 2 diabetes

Management of insulin treated diabetes during surgery

The chief principle of diabetic management through any crisis in which patients cannot eat or drink for any reason is to continue insulin administration. The best method is to give the insulin by continuous intravenous infusion either by infusion pump or directly from the drip bag.

For operations in which a patient is likely to be maintained on a drip for more than 12 hours a regimen is needed which can be continued for an indefinite period. Again there are two methods of administering the insulin: a variable rate infusion using a pump, or if this is not available, a glucose insulin-infusion. **Note**:

- The rate of intravenous infusion must depend on the clinical state of the patient with regard to the volume depletion, cardiac failure, age, etc.
- Potassium replacement is required.
- If the blood glucose is persistently above 10 mmol/l the infusion should be changed to 0·9% saline.
- Blood glucose should be monitored every one to two hours during surgery and regularly postoperatively.
- Try to maintain the blood glucose concentration in a safe range—6·0-12 mmol/l.
- Regular (at least daily) electrolyte measurements are required.

After recovery: changing to subcutaneous insulin
Once the patient starts to eat and drink conversion back to subcutaneous insulin injections is undertaken as follows.

- Always change to subcutaneous insulin before breakfast and never in the evening so that adequate supervision can be assured.
- Stop the insulin pump 30 minutes after the first subcutaneous insulin injection.
- Insulin regimen and dose: if the previous regimen is known then this should be given; if the patient is still in bed or unwell the total dose may need to be 10 to 20% more than usual. If the patient was not previously taking insulin, predicting the requirement is not easy and the amount needs adjustment from day to day. Initially use insulin 30-40 units daily in divided doses given four times daily.

Patients with hyperglycaemia often relapse after conversion back to subcutaneous insulin. When this happens there are three possible approaches.

- Give additional doses of soluble insulin at any of the four injection times (before meals or bedtime).
- Add an intravenous insulin infusion temporarily while continuing the subcutaneous regimen until the blood glucose concentration is satisfactory.
- Revert completely to the intravenous regimen, especially if the patient is unwell.

Surgery in Type 2 diabetes
Management of diabetic patients treated with diet or oral hypoglycaemic agents is more straightforward, so long as the diabetes is well controlled.

If the random blood glucose value is less than 12 mmol/l:

- omit the tablet on the day of surgery
- check the blood glucose concentration before and soon after the operation; if the blood glucose value is more than 12 mmol/l start soluble insulin.

If the diabetes is poorly controlled (random blood glucose greater than 12 mmol/l) the patient should be started on

---

Dextrose drip and variable rate insulin infusion
(1) Give normal insulin on the night before the operation
(2) Early on the day of operation start an infusion of 10% dextrose, add 20 mmol potassium chloride to each litre, and run at a *constant* rate appropriate to the patient's fluid requirement, usually 100 ml/h
(3) Make up a solution of soluble insulin 1 unit/ml saline in a syringe and infuse intravenously by a line piggybacked to the intravenous drip by using a syringe pump. The infusion rate should normally be as shown in regimen 1, but in resistant cases use regimen 2 or 3

Blood glucose	Soluble insulin infusion rate		
	Regimen 1	Regimen 2	Regimen 3
<4 mmol/l	0·5 unit/h	1 unit/h	2 unit/h
4-10 mmol/l	2 unit/h	4 unit/h	8 unit/h
10-15 mmol/l	4 unit/h	8 unit/h	16 unit/h
15-20 mmol/l	6 unit/h	12 unit/h	24 unit/h
>20 mmol/l	Review		

Blood glucose is measured preoperatively and then two hourly until stable, then six hourly

Regimen 1 is satisfactory for most cases; very severely ill patients, shocked patients, and those receiving steroids, salbutamol, or dopexamine infusions may need higher dose infusions, such as regimens 2 or 3, occasionally even more.

Do not stop the insulin infusion since intravenous insulin lasts for only a few minutes

Only if the patient becomes frankly hypoglycaemic (blood glucose <2·0 mmol/l) should insulin be stopped for up to 30 minutes

---

Glucose-insulin infusion
(1) Give normal insulin on the night before the operation
(2) Begin an infusion of 10% dextrose containing 20 mmol/l potassium chloride and soluble insulin 15 units/l. Run it at a rate appropriate to the patient's fluid requirements, usually 100 ml/h. Adjust insulin dose as follows

Blood glucose	Soluble insulin infusion
<4 mmol/l	15 unit/l
4-10 mmol/l	30 unit/l
10-15 mmol/l	40 unit/l
15-20 mmol/l	60 unit/l
>20 mmol/l	Review

Blood glucose is measured two hourly until stable, then six hourly

---

Surgery in Type 2 diabetes
- Omit usual treatment
- Use insulin if diabetic control deteriorates
- Maintain blood glucose chart

insulin before the operation, using one of the regimens described on the previous page.

Management of insulin treated diabetes during day surgery
Patients with insulin treated diabetes requiring an anaesthetic for relatively minor operations or investigative procedures (for example, barium radiological examinations, cystoscopy, endoscopy, etc.) can be treated as day cases without hospital admission provided that:

- the procedure is undertaken in the morning first on the list (if the procedure is performed first on an afternoon list, a light breakfast is taken after half the normal insulin dose, followed by regular blood glucose monitoring)
- the procedure does not exceed approximately one hour in duration
- the patient will be able to eat and drink within one hour of the procedure
- the patient is able to self-monitor blood glucose and adjust insulin appropriately.

The blood glucose should be rechecked before discharge. If significant problems with diabetes control persist, then hospital admission may be required after all.

Instructions for management of insulin treated diabetes in day surgery
- The procedure should be performed after an overnight fast
- Insulin is taken on the previous evening as usual
- Insulin and breakfast are omitted on the morning of the procedure
- The blood glucose must be measured before leaving home and again before the procedure is commenced.
- If the blood glucose is less than 6·0 mmol/l a 10% dextrose drip is needed
- Within one hour after completion of the procedure, the normal morning insulin dose should be administered followed by appropriate food and fluid giving the equivalent amount of carbohydrate to the usual breakfast

The photograph of blood glucose and ketone meter is with permission from MediSense.

10   Diabetic complications: cause and prevention

Introduction

Patients with long-standing diabetes may develop complications affecting the eyes, kidneys or nerves (microvascular complications) or major arteries. The major arteries are affected in people with diabetes, causing a substantial increase in both in coronary artery disease and strokes as well as peripheral vascular disease. The greatest risk of large vessel disease occurs in those diabetic patients who develop proteinuria or microalbuminuria, which are associated with widespread vascular damage. These complications are often discovered at presentation in Type 2 diabetic patients who must have had diabetes for many years before it has been diagnosed. Issues concerning macrovascular complications are described in chapter 17.

During the last two decades, there has been a considerable increase in understanding the mechanisms underlying the development of the long-term diabetic microvascular complications (retinopathy, nephropathy, and neuropathy) and macrovascular disease, accompanied by major developments in preventing them. The United Kingdom Prospective Diabetes Survey (UKPDS) in particular demonstrated quantitatively the long-term harmful effects of hyperglycaemia and hypertension in the development of both microvascular and macrovascular complications in Type 2 diabetes. Both UKPDS and the Diabetes Complications and Control Trial (DCCT) of Type 1 diabetes demonstrated the benefits of optimal control.

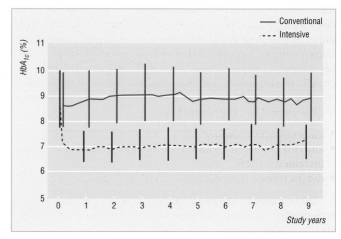

HbA$_{1c}$ values during 9 years in the DCCT study of Type 1 diabetes, showing steady levels in intensively and conventionally controlled groups

Causes and prevention of complications

Major advances in recent years have resulted in an actual decrease of some complications, notably nephropathy. Primary prevention of diabetic complications, together with retardation of their progression, is now possible, chiefly by tight control of the diabetes and of hypertension, together with reduction of other "risk factors" detailed in chapter 17. Even when the complications are established, their progression leading to serious damage can be delayed.

Although many attempts have been made to develop specific pharmacological agents to alter the course of diabetic complications, and although many trials are in progress at the present time, none have proved unequivocally successful and none are licensed. There is at present intense interest in and optimism for the use of protein kinase-C inhibitors.

Two major studies
DCCT: a multicentre study of 1441 Type 1 diabetic patients in the United States examining the effects of tight control on the development of microvascular complications, terminated after nine years because of highly significant benefits reported in 1993. The benefits on the microvascular complications were considerable.

UKPDS: a multicentre study of 5102 Type 2 diabetic patients co-ordinated from Oxford, assessed both the harmful effects of persistent hyperglycaemia and hypertension on the development of microvascular and macrovascular complications, and also demonstrated the

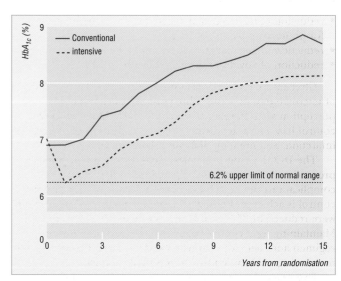

HbA$_{1c}$ values during 15 years of the UKPDS study of Type 2 diabetes showing progressive deterioration of both intensively and conventionally controlled groups

benefits of 10 years of better, compared with less satisfactory, control of both glycaemia and blood pressure reported in 1998. Benefits were achieved regardless of the drugs used to reach the required standards of either blood glucose or blood pressure control.

The long-term effects of treatment in the two studies are shown in the two figures demonstrating the stable control in Type 1 diabetes (DCCT) compared with the deteriorating control in Type 2 diabetes as the disease progresses (UKPDS).

Persistent hyperglycaemia
Over many years this is the principal underlying cause of the microvascular complications of diabetes. It is also an independent risk factor for the development of macrovascular coronary artery disease and cataract formation. The UKPDS showed precisely the increasing hazard in relation to continuously rising HbA_{1c} levels, without any specific threshold point, and then demonstrated the benefits of tight control. Once complications are established additional factors, notably hypertension, may accelerate their progression (for further details see chapters on specific complications).

For every 1% increase in HbA_{1c}:

- microvascular complications increased by 37%
- any end point (micro and macrovascular) related to diabetes increased by 21%
- deaths related to diabetes increased by 21%.

(Microvascular complications are here defined as retinopathy requiring photocoagulation, vitreous haemorrhage, and fatal or non-fatal renal failure.)

The progression of neuropathy assessed in a group of Type 1 diabetic patients in a prospective 14-year study conducted in Dusseldorf has also shown clearly that the decline of numerous measurements of nerve function occurs almost exclusively in those with poor glycaemic control.

The effect of better blood glucose control on the microvascular complications was as follows:

- reduction of microvascular complications (chiefly the need for photocoagulation) by 25%
- reduction of any diabetes end point by 12%
- reduction of any diabetes related death by 10%.

Glycaemic control was also shown to reduce the evolution of microalbuminuria after nine years, and the loss of vibration perception after 15 years of the study. Tight blood glucose control had a non-significant effect on reduction of myocardial infarction, and none on diabetes related mortality.

The DCCT (Type 1 diabetes) demonstrated that primary prevention and retardation of progression of diabetic complications can be achieved over a decade if tight diabetic control is achieved. Retinopathy, nephropathy, and neuropathy were reduced by 35-70% if HbA_{1c} was maintained around 7%. Maintaining tight control requires optimisation of insulin regimen and diet (see chapters 5 and 6), careful blood glucose monitoring, and substantial professional support.

Five years after termination of the DCCT, the EPIC study showed that, despite lapse of the earlier tight blood glucose control, the benefits with regard to amelioration of complications persisted.

Hypertension
This is the principal underlying risk factor for the development of coronary artery disease leading to myocardial infarction, and increases the risk of strokes and heart failure as well.

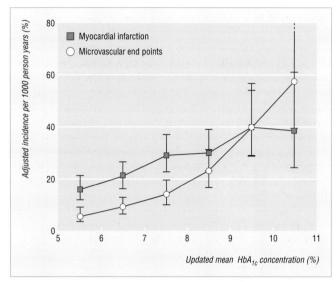

Incidence rates and 95% confidence intervals for myocardial infarction and microvascular complications by category of updated mean HbA_{1c} values, adjusted for age, sex, and ethnic group, expressed for white men aged 50-54 years at diagnosis and with mean duration of Type 2 diabetes of 10 years (UKPDS)

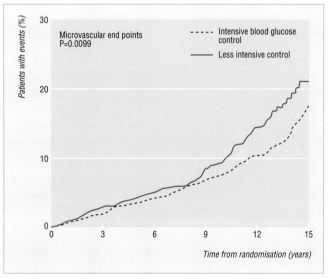

Kaplan-Meier plot of aggregate microvascular end points resulting from intensive and less intensive blood glucose control in patients with Type 2 diabetes in UKPDS. Microvascular disease here includes renal failure, death from renal failure, retinal photocoagulation, or vitreous haemorrhage

ABC of Diabetes

It also exacerbates the progression of retinopathy, the evolution of proteinuria, and probably the deterioration of nerve function as well.

The UKPDS (Type 2 diabetes) has shown that for every 10 mm Hg increase in systolic blood pressure:

- any complication related to diabetes is increased by 12%
- deaths related to diabetes are increased by 15%
- myocardial infarction is increased by 11%
- microvascular complications are increased by 13%.

By achieving a mean blood pressure of 144/82, representing a reduction of systolic blood pressure of 10 mm Hg compared with the less intensively treated group, microvascular end points (chiefly the need for photocoagulation) were reduced by 37%, and risk of vision declining by three lines on the Snellen chart was reduced by 47%, chiefly by protection from the development of macular disease.

Better control of blood pressure also resulted in a 32% reduction in deaths related to diabetes, and a 44% reduction in strokes; there was a non-significant reduction in myocardial infarction.

Further details on the benefits of good blood pressure control in general and on established nephropathy in particular are described in chapters 16 and 17.

Smoking
This exacerbates all the complications of diabetes, both microvascular and macrovascular.

Dyslipidaemias
These increase the propensity to macrovascular disease: targets for control are described in chapter 17.

The presence of the above factors in combination additively increases the risks of developing complications.

Targets for control and reduction of risk factors
Blood glucose
The facility for patients to measure their own blood glucose empowers them to achieve optimal control by their own interventions. The aims are as follows:

- Type 1 diabetes: achieve preprandial blood glucose readings mainly in the range 4·5-7·7 mmol/l, postprandial readings in the range 6·0-9·0 mmol/l, and 7·0-9·0 mmol/l at bedtime, and preferably never below 4·0 mmol/l to avoid blunting of hypoglycaemic awareness.
- Type 2 diabetes: fasting <5·5 mmol/l;
  postprandial <9·0 mmol/l.

Glycated haemoglobin
Aim for an HbA$_{1c}$<6·5% (normal value 4·0-6·0%) as an ideal, since values >7% are increasingly associated with development of all microvascular and macrovascular complications, and reduction of HbA$_{1c}$ has been shown to diminish microvascular complications substantially (see below). Values up to 8% are acceptable in those who cannot readily achieve the ideal (and there are many). When HbA$_{1c}$ values exceed 9%, additional education and counselling should be attempted although even then patients may not succeed, and some show no inclination to do so.

Blood pressure
Targets for control are described in chapter 17.

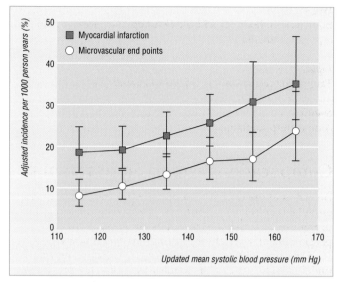

Incidence rates (95% confidence interval) of myocardial infarction and microvascular end points by category of updated mean systolic blood pressure, adjusted for age, sex, and ethnic group expressed for white men aged 50-54 years at diagnosis and mean duration of Type 2 diabetes of 10 years (UKPDS)

> The benefits of controlling glycaemia required persistently good control over a decade; benefits of successful blood pressure control were witnessed after approximately 4 to 5 years

Targets for glycaemic control suggested by the European Diabetes Policy Group

	Low risk	Arterial risk	Microvascular risk
HbA$_{1c}$ %	≤6·5	>6·5	>7·5
Venous plasma glucose			
Fasting/preprandial			
mmol/l	≤6·0	>6·0	≥7·0
mg/dl	<110	≥110	≥126
*Self-monitored blood glucose**			
Fasting/preprandial			
mmol/l	≤5·5	>5·5	>6·0
mg/dl	<100	≥100	≥110
Postprandial or peak			
mmol/l	<7·5	≥7·5	>9·0
mg/dl	<135	≥135	>160

*Fasting capillary blood glucose is about 1·0 mmol/l (18 mg/dl) lower than venous plasma blood glucose. Postprandial capillary blood glucose is about the same as venous plasma blood glucose

Weight
Body mass index < 25 is ideal; 27 acceptable; greater than 30 represents obesity.

Lipids
Targets for control are described in chapter 17.

Smoking
Aim: to stop smoking.

Complications screening programme

Detection of the earliest signs of diabetic complications is an essential requirement of diabetes care leading to early preventive and treatment strategies which can abort progression of some of the most serious consequences.

Screening is ideally performed as a structured service undertaken by nurses and technicians outside the process of professional consultation, which should be informed by printed results from the screening programme. Screening should be performed at onset and then annually, from the onset of diabetes in all diabetic patients. Complications in Type 1 diabetes, however, are unlikely to develop during the first five years after diagnosis, so that the complete annual screening protocol can be deferred for a short time. The screening programme can be performed wherever appropriate facilities exist. Once complications are present and established, more frequent screening or treatment, or both may be needed.

Eye screening requires specialist equipment and is often undertaken as a community responsibility, and there are strong representations that there should be a national screening programme. Detection and prevention of foot problems linked to delivery of adequate community podiatry services is also crucial and highly effective in preventing serious foot disorders.

The annual complications screening programme
This comprises:

- weight (height): body mass index
- blood pressure
- eye examination (visual acuity, fundoscopy, and photography)
- foot examination:
  check for deformities, abrasions and ulcers
  sensation (monofilament tests, and other sensory modalities if available, see pages 52 and 63)
  palpate foot pulses
- blood tests: HbA$_{1c}$; lipid profile; creatinine
- urine tests: strip tests for proteinuria or microalbuminuria (if either of these are positive, total 24 hour proteinuria or the albumin creatinine ratio (ACR) should be measured, preferably on an early morning urine sample)
- assessment of smoking status.

Other complications

Necrobiosis lipoidica diabeticorum
Necrobiosis is an uncommon and unsightly blemish of the skin which chiefly affects diabetic women. It is unrelated to microvascular complications. The shin is the most common site. The lesions show rather atrophic skin at the centre with obviously dilated capillaries (telangiectasis) and a slightly raised pinkish rim; ulceration sometimes occurs. The lesions are indolent and rarely resolve. There is no effective treatment although steroid applications and even injection have been attempted.

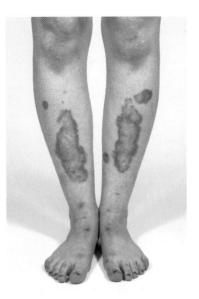

Necrobiosis lipoidica diabeticorum

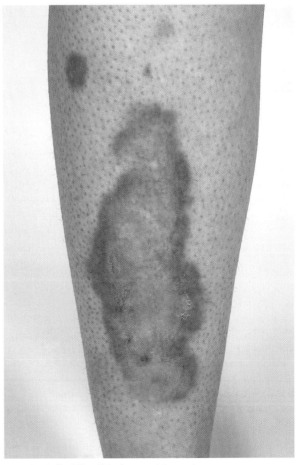

Necrobiosis lipoidica diabeticorum (close up)

Cheiroarthropathy

The development of tight, waxy skin, probably as a result of glucose related alteration of collagen structure, leads to some limitation of joint mobility. A relatively common yet symptomless consequence of these skin changes is the development of some fixed curvature of the fingers which may typically be seen in some patients with long-term diabetes. Those affected are unable to place the palm of the hand on a flat surface. The characteristic appearance is shown in the illustration on the right.

The figure showing the HbA_{1c} values during 9 years in the DCCT study of Type 1 diabetes is adapted from DCCT investigators. *New Engl J Med* 1993;329:977-86. The HbA_{1c} values during 15 years of UKPDS study of Type 2 diabetes and the Kaplan-Meier plot of aggregate microvascular end points are adapted from Diabetes Control and Complications Research Group. *New Engl J Med* 1993;329:977-86. The figures showing incidence rates and 95% confidence interval for myocardial infarction and microvascular complication by category of updated mean HbA_{1c} values and mean systolic blood pressure are adapted from UKPDS. *BMJ* 2000;321:405-17. The table showing targets for glycaemic control is adapted from European Diabetes Policy Group *Diabetic Med* 1999;16:716-30.

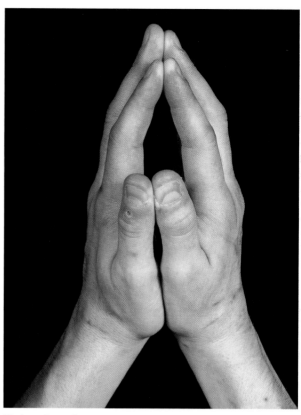

Cheiroarthropathy

11   Retinopathy

Blindness is one of the most feared complications of diabetes, but also one of the most preventable. Diabetes is the commonest cause of blindness in people aged 30 to 69 years. Twenty years after the onset of diabetes almost all patients with Type 1 diabetes and over 60% of patients with Type 2 diabetes will have some degree of retinopathy, and even at the time of diagnosis of Type 2 diabetes, approximately one-quarter of patients already have established background retinopathy. As treatment is now available to prevent blindness in the majority of cases, it is essential to identify patients with retinopathy before their vision is affected.

Classification of retinopathy

Diabetic retinopathy is due to microangiopathy affecting the retinal precapillary arterioles, capillaries, and venules. Damage is caused by both microvascular leakage due to break down of the inner blood-retinal barrier and microvascular occlusion. These two pathological mechanisms can be distinguished from each other by fluorescein angiography, which is the "gold standard" for assessing diabetic retinopathy.

Background retinopathy
Microaneurysms are small saccular pouches possibly caused by local distension of capillary walls. They are often the first clinically detectable sign of retinopathy, and appear as small red dots commonly temporal to the macula.

   Haemorrhages may occur within the compact middle layers of the retina, and appear as "dot" or "blot" haemorrhages, or

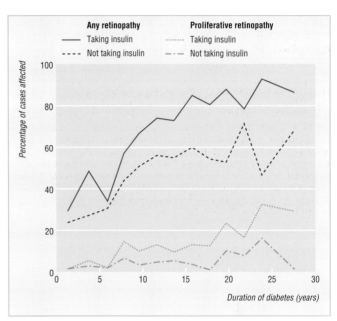

Frequency of retinopathy (any degree) and proliferative retinopathy by duration of diabetes in people receiving or not receiving insulin, and who were diagnosed to have diabetes at or after 30 years of age

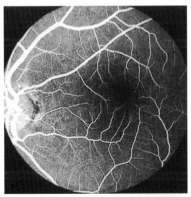

Fluorescein angiogram showing normal eye

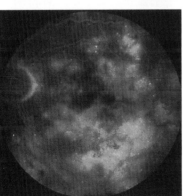

Fluorescein angiogram showing capillary leakage with macular oedema

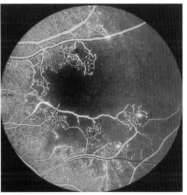

Fluorescein angiogram showing capillary closure

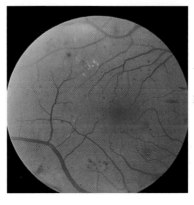

Microaneurysms, haemorrhages, and exudates

rarely, in the superficial nerve fibre layer where they appear as "flame shaped" haemorrhages (the latter better recognised as related to severe hypertension).

Hard exudates are yellow lipid deposits with relatively discrete margins. They commonly occur at the edges of microvascular leakage, and may form a "circinate" pattern around a leaking microaneurysm. They may coalesce to form extensive sheets of exudate. Vision is affected when hard exudates encroach upon the macula.

Retinal oedema is due to microvascular leakage and indicates breakdown of the inner blood-retinal barrier. It appears clinically as greyish areas of retinal thickening, and may assume a petal-shaped cystoid appearance at the macula, where it may cause marked visual deterioration.

Clinically significant macular oedema (CSMO) requires treatment. It is defined as any one of the following:

- retinal oedema within 500 μm (one-third of a disc diameter) of the fovea
- hard exudates within 500 μm of the fovea, if associated with adjacent retinal thickening
- retinal oedema that is one disc diameter (1500 μm) or larger, any part of which is within one disc diameter of the fovea.

Twenty percent of eyes with untreated CSMO will suffer significant visual loss in two years compared with 8% of treated eyes.

Pre-proliferative retinopathy
Retinal ischaemia due to microvascular occlusion may lead to neovascular proliferation. Signs of ischaemia include:

- cotton wool spots, which appear as white patches with rather feathery margins and represent nerve fibre layer microinfarcts; they become highly significant when there are more than five
- large dark "blot" haemorrhages
- venous beading and looping
- intraretinal microvascular abnormalities (IRMA).

Proliferative retinopathy
New vessel formation may occur at the optic disc (NVD) or elsewhere on the retina (NVE). Disc new vessels are particularly threatening to vision and if allowed to progress commonly lead to vitreous haemorrhage. If untreated, 26% of eyes with "high-risk" and neovascular proliferation on the disc will progress to severe visual loss within two years. With laser treatment this is reduced to 11%.

Advanced eye disease
In advanced proliferative diabetic retinopathy, progressive fibrovascular proliferation leads to blindness due to vitreous haemorrhage and traction retinal detachment. Rubeosis iridis and neovascular glaucoma occur when new vessels form on the

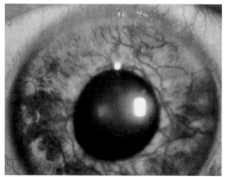

Rubeosis iridis

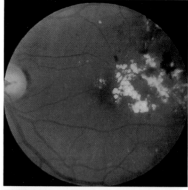

Exudative maculopathy

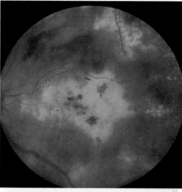

Exudative maculopathy

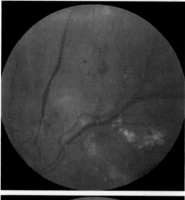

Pre-proliferative retinopathy with venous bleeding, cotton wool spots and some hard exudates

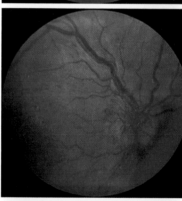

Disc new vessels (NVD)

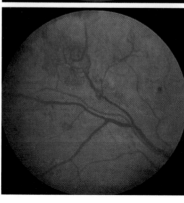

New vessels elsewhere (NVE)

iris and in the anterior chamber drainage angle, leading to a most painful blind eye which occasionally requires enucleation.

Blindness in diabetic patients

Vision-threatening retinopathy is usually due mainly to neovascularisation in Type 1 diabetes and maculopathy in Type 2 diabetes. In North America, 3·6% of patients with Type 1 diabetes and 1·6% of patients with Type 2 diabetes are legally blind. In England and Wales about 1000 diabetic patients are registered as blind or partially sighted each year, with diabetic retinopathy being the commonest cause of blindness in the working population.

Vitreous haemorrhage occurs suddenly and painlessly. The blood usually clears over the following weeks, but the underlying proliferative retinopathy causes repeated haemorrhages and progressive visual loss in most cases if it is not treated. Retinal detachment resulting from contracting fibrous bonds sometimes causes blindness.

Maculopathy: Macular disease has three causes in diabetic patients—exudative maculopathy, retinal oedema, and ischaemia. Deterioration of vision in these situations is often insidious, it can to some extent be prevented by appropriate laser treatment, but once vision has been lost it cannot be restored. Ischaemic maculopathy due to loss of perifoveal capillaries may cause severe visual loss and is very difficult to treat.

Cataract: Lens opacities or cataract develop earlier in diabetic patients and often progress more rapidly.

Primary open-angle glaucoma has an increased prevalence in diabetic patients compared with the general population.

Prevention of blindness

The presence of retinopathy must be actively sought by physicians because, if detected early enough, blindness can be prevented in many cases by treatment with laser photocoagulation. The indications for laser treatment are:

- NVD or NVE; advanced pre-proliferative changes
- clinically significant macular oedema as defined above
- encroachment of hard exudates towards the fovea.

Chronic vitreous haemorrhage which precludes a view of the retina can be treated by vitrectomy and endolaser. Tractional retinal detachment can be managed by vitrectomy with the use of heavy liquids and silicone oil. Restoration of visual acuity can be impressive, but is dependent on the underlying condition of the retina itself.

Clinical examination of the eyes and screening

(For further details on screening see page 45)

Visual acuity and retinal examination should be performed annually on all diabetic patients after 12 years of age, or more often if advancing changes are observed. Vision-threatening retinopathy rarely occurs in Type 1 diabetes in the first five years after diagnosis or before puberty. However, more than one-quarter of Type 2 diabetic patients have been found to have retinopathy at diagnosis, and screening should start immediately.

Visual acuity should be checked annually, or more often if significant retinopathy is present or if it has changed

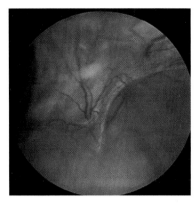
Advanced eye diseae—Retinitis proliferans

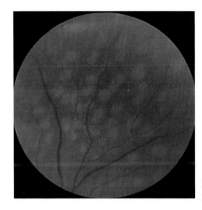
Recent argon laser photocoagulation

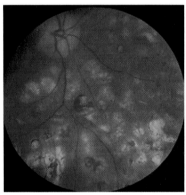
Longstanding photocoagulation scars

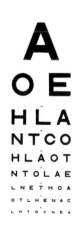

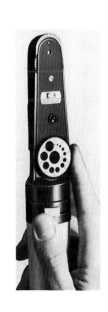

unexpectedly. This should be done with patients wearing their spectacles or through a "pinhole" if they are not.

Retinal examination. Routine fundal examination should be performed on all diabetic patients, using fundoscopy or retinal photography or preferably both. The pupils should be dilated and the fundus examined in a darkened room. Tropicamide 1% (Mydriacil) eye drops are recommended as they have a short duration of action of just two to three hours. There is no reason to avoid pupillary dilatation in patients being treated for chronic open-angle glaucoma, although those on treatment for closed-angle glaucoma must not undergo pupillary dilatation.

Once background retinopathy is present the patients should be examined every six to 12 months or more often if there is any change of visual acuity, and referred to an ophthalmologist when indicated (see box). Pregnant patients require more frequent follow up as retinopathy may progress rapidly during pregnancy (see page 78).

Screening methods

Conventional examination, using an ophthalmoscope in a darkened room with the pupil dilated is a minimum requirement. Observers must be well trained, but even consultant ophthalmologists do not achieve the required 80% sensitivity.

Retinal photography through dilated pupils. The preferred method now uses digital photography which yields suitable images which can be electronically stored, making them easily available for consultation, review, and teaching. Conventional colour photographs also provide good images, whereas the quality of Polaroid photographs is less than ideal.

It would be ideal to provide both conventional funduscopic and photographic screening procedures, and there is already some evidence that the combined screening procedure reduces the failure rate. A national screening programme has been proposed and has already been adopted in Wales.

The blind diabetic patient

Blind registration is available for those patients with visual acuity of less than 3/60 in their better eye or gross field defects, affording some financial help and social service support. Patients with a visual acuity of less than 6/60 in their better eye are eligible for registration as partially sighted. They must be registered by an ophthalmologist using the BD8 form. Printing in braille is valuable but many diabetic patients have impaired fine sensation in their fingertips, making it difficult for them to read it. Insulin "pens", in which palpable clicks correspond to units of insulin are valuable for blind patients.

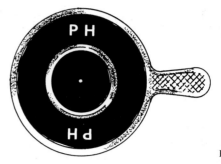

Pin hole

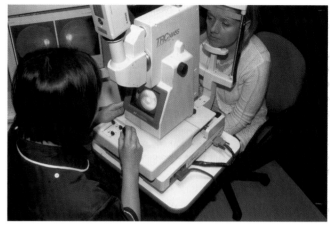

Digital camera used for retinal photography

Indications for referral to an ophthalmologist

- Reduced visual acuity from any cause
- Presence of proliferative or pre-proliferative changes
- Presence of clinically significant macular oedema
- Presence of hard exudates near the macula
- Presence of any form of progressing or extensive diabetic retinopathy especially when the lesions are near the macula

The figure showing frequency of retinopathy is adapted from Pickup JC, Williams G, eds. *Textbook of diabetes*, 2nd ed, Oxford: Blackwell Scientific Publications, 1997.

12 Peripheral neuropathies

Diabetic neuropathies constitute a diverse group of conditions. The commonest is a diffuse polyneuropathy which damages distal peripheral nerves (chiefly affecting the feet), together with the autonomic nervous system. The dying back of axons is associated with segmental demyelination. Polyneuropathy is a classic diabetic complication developing mainly in those with poor diabetic control, progressing (albeit at very variable rates) as the duration of diabetes lengthens and often, but not always, associated with other long-term diabetic complications. In contrast, mononeuropathies and acute painful neuropathies run a well-defined course from the relatively acute onset to almost complete recovery in six to 18 months. These reversible neuropathies, which may be the reason for initial presentation of diabetes, can occur after any duration of diabetes, are commoner in Type 2 diabetic men, and are not necessarily associated with other diabetic complications.

Pressure neuropathies are commoner in those with diabetes and include carpal tunnel syndrome (median nerve), ulnar neuropathy, and rarely foot drop (lateral popliteal nerve).

> **Diabetic neuropathies**
>
> **Progress**
> - Diffuse polyneuropathy
>   Symmetrical sensory neuropathy
>   Autonomic neuropathy
>
> **Recover**
> - Mononeuropathies
>   Proximal motor (femoral) neuropathy
>   Radiculopathies (especially truncal)
>   Cranial nerve palsies
> - Acute painful neuropathies

Symmetrical sensory neuropathy

Diffuse neuropathy affects peripheral nerves symmetrically, chiefly those of the feet and legs. It is almost always sensory, though motor involvement causing weakness, and wasting does occur rarely. Peripheral neuropathy is common in long-standing diabetic patients, but in Type 2 diabetic patients it may already be present at the onset of diabetes. Progression of neuropathy is reduced by good control of diabetes over many years. The potential of pharmacological agents to alter the course of neuropathy has been extensively studied, but so far none of the drugs investigated has demonstrated convincing clinically significant benefit.

Neuropathy is usually symptomless and therefore a hazard to the unwary patient, who is at risk of foot injury and infection. In more advanced neuropathies the patient is aware of sensory loss; numbness (and in some, a sensation of coldness) may progressively worsen until there is almost complete anaesthesia below the knee associated with proprioceptive loss which makes patients feel quite unsafe, but this is not common. Paraesthesiae are quite often described by patients: they range from a persistent minor inconvenience to a source of considerable discomfort and even pain needing medication to alleviate the symptoms. Management of painful neuropathy is described on page 57.

Neurological examination almost always reveals absent ankle reflexes, and only rarely absent knee reflexes. Diminished light-touch and vibration perception are common and by careful examination can be shown to occur at an almost identical level in both legs, hence the description of "stocking" neuropathy. Some patients demonstrate a highly selective form of sensory impairment with gross loss of pain and thermal sensation (accompanied by severely abnormal autonomic function tests) while light-touch and vibration perception remain almost intact. Such a dissociated sensory loss can cause some confusion in the clinical assessment of neuropathy. Impairment of joint position sense is extremely unusual except in the most advanced cases. Further details of clinical sensory assessment are described on page 63.

Diabetic neuropathies

	Recover	Progress
	Mononeuropathies/ painful neuropathies	Sensory/autonomic neuropathy
Onset	acute	gradual
Duration of diabetes mellitus	any	long standing
Other complications	none	often
Sex	M > F	M = F*
Diabetes mellitus	Type 2 > Type 1	Type 1 = Type 2*

*Symptomatic autonomic neuropathy occurs chiefly in female Type 1 diabetic patients

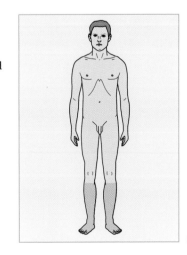

Symmetrical sensory neuropathy

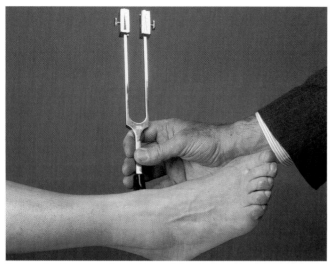

Testing vibration perception at the medial malleolus with a Rydell Seifer quantitative tuning fork

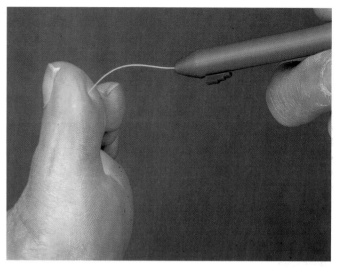

Testing light-touch sensation with a monofilament

Neuropathy and the hands

Diabetic neuropathy rarely causes symptoms in the hands, and when it does the disease is already advanced in the feet and legs. Numbness and clumsiness of the fingers are thus very unusual and more likely to be due to some other neurological disorder. Impairment of sensation is, however, enough to prevent blind diabetics from reading braille. Paraesthesiae and numbness in the fingers, especially at night, are usually due to carpal tunnel syndrome, which is commoner than in non-diabetics. It is easily and effectively relieved by minor surgery performed under local anaesthetic without admission to hospital.

Interosseous muscle wasting, especially of the first dorsal interosseous, is often seen. It is usually due to ulnar nerve compression at the elbow, and typical sensory defects in the fourth and fifth fingers are detectable. It causes little disability and there is no satisfactory treatment. Patients are advised not to lean on their elbows, thereby avoiding further damage to the ulnar nerve.

Neuropathy and the feet

Reduced sensation in the feet may result in unnoticed trauma from ill-fitting shoes, nails or stones when walking barefoot, or burns from hot water bottles or sitting too close to a fire. Self-inflicted wounds from crude attempts at chiropody are dangerous because they often become infected. Proprietary corn cures which contain salicylic acid can cause ulceration, sepsis and necrosis, and should never be used. Diabetic foot disorders are described in chapter 15.

Features of neuropathy of the hands

- Inability to read braille
- Carpal tunnel compression
- Ulnar nerve compression

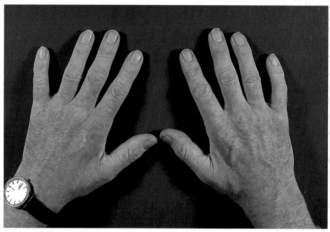

Interosseous muscle wasting

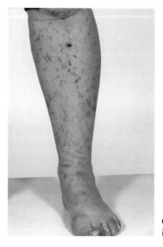

Cat scratches on a neuropathic, insensitive leg

13 Autonomic neuropathy

Diffuse damage to both parasympathetic and sympathetic nerves, probably developing in that order, is common in diabetic patients with diffuse peripheral neuropathy. Fortunately the disabling symptoms which result are not common, and even when they do occur some of them, especially diarrhoea, vomiting, and postural hypotension, are curiously intermittent.

Gastrointestinal system

Diarrhoea
This is a catastrophic watery diarrhoea with severe nocturnal exacerbations and faecal incontinence, preceded momentarily by characteristic abdominal rumblings. Malabsorption does not normally occur. The symptoms are intermittent, with normal bowel actions in between, and sometimes even constipation. These features persist for months or years, rarely disappearing altogether. The diagnosis is made, firstly, by excluding other causes of diarrhoea such as coeliac disease or pancreatic malfunction, and secondly, by establishing the presence of peripheral and autonomic neuropathy. The diarrhoea may be treated with any antidiarrhoeal agent, the best of which is codeine phosphate. Tetracycline in two or three doses of 250 mg has a dramatic effect in about half of patients; it should only be used at the onset of an attack. Some authorities suggest the use of tetracycline or metronidazole for two to three weeks but long-term antibiotics are not indicated. Clonidine can be tried but is of little value; octreotide can be effective but side effects are common.

Gastroparesis
Diminished gastric motility and delayed stomach emptying sometimes occur in diabetic patients with autonomic neuropathy, but rarely cause symptoms. Intermittent vomiting may occur, and in exceptional cases it is intractable. The diagnosis is established by the presence of a gastric splash, impaired gastric emptying on investigation by isotopic techniques, and screening during barium studies; endoscopy and other investigations are needed to exclude other gastric disorders. Any antiemetic can be useful, including metoclopramide or domperidone. Erythromycin acting as a motilin agonist has been used but is only of value when used intravenously. In the very rare cases of intractable vomiting, percutaneous endoscopic jejunostomy can help, and even more rarely radical surgery by two-thirds gastrectomy with Roux-en-Y loop may be required and can succeed.

Cardiovascular system: postural hypotension

Postural hypotension is defined by a fall in systolic blood pressure on standing of more than 20 mm Hg. Development of symptoms depends both on the actual fall of blood pressure (usually greater than 30 mm Hg) and on the actual systolic blood pressure when standing, which becomes impossible if it is less than 70 mm Hg. When assessing postural hypotension, the blood pressure should be taken with the patient lying down,

Clinical features of autonomic neuropathy

Gastrointestinal
- Diarrhoea
- Gastroparesis

Cardiovascular
- Postural hypotension
- Persistent tachycardia
- High foot blood flow
- Vascular medial calcification

Genitourinary
- Erectile dysfunction
- Neurogenic bladder

Sweating
- Gustatory sweating
- Dry feet

Respiratory
- Depressed cough reflex
- Respiratory arrests
- ? Deaths from respiratory arrests

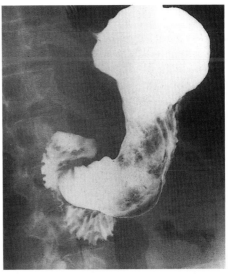

Radiograph showing food retention caused by gastroparesis

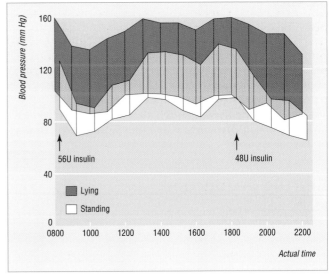

Insulin exacerbates postural hypotension

and the standing reading taken over approximately three minutes during which the time blood pressure continues to fall.

Treatment is only needed if symptoms occur and if they are troublesome, which is rare. Patients should stop drugs which might aggravate hypotension (notably tranquillisers, antidepressants, and diuretics), sleep with the head of the bed raised, and wear full length elastic stockings. The best results are obtained from measures which increase plasma volume, namely a high salt intake and fludrocortisone (increasing the dose slowly from 0·1 to 0·4 mg). Treatment failures are common, and the oedema which results from treatment may be disagreeable. Successful treatment has been reported with indomethacin; a combination of fludrocortisone, flurbiprofen, and ephedrine may help. Midodrine is an α agonist which is also of value and available on a named patient basis.

Treatment of hypotension
- Stop drugs that may aggravate hypotension
- Sleep with head of bed raised
- Wear full length elastic stockings
- Appropriate medication

Gustatory sweating

Facial sweating (including scalp, neck, and shoulders) which occurs while eating tasty food, notably cheese, is a common symptom of autonomic neuropathy. Once present, it seems to persist indefinitely, although amelioration after renal transplantation occurs for no known reason.

When it becomes a severe embarrassment with sweat rolling down the face and chest at every meal, it can be effectively treated with an anticholinergic agent, namely propantheline bromide, although side effects are common, or by a topical application of glypyrronium powder. The cream should be applied on alternate days to the areas affected by sweating, avoiding contact with the mouth, nose, and eyes. The area should not be washed for four hours after application. Systemic absorption is low and the only contraindication is narrow-angle glaucoma, as there is the possibility of accidental direct instillation into the eye. Although recommended to be given on alternate days, many patients prefer to use it only on social occasions.

Respiratory arrests

Transient respiratory arrest occurs sometimes if susceptible neuropathic patients are given any agent which depresses respiration, notably anaesthetics or powerful analgesics such as morphine and its derivatives. These patients must be monitored carefully even during minor surgery. Rare unexplained deaths in patients with established autonomic neuropathy may be due to respiratory arrest.

Neurogenic bladder

Urinary retention is a serious and usually late complication of autonomic neuropathy. Apart from the discomfort, intractable urinary infections may develop. The diagnosis of bladder retention is now simple using ultrasound techniques. Cystoscopy may be needed to exclude other causes of bladder neck obstruction. Treatment is now by self catheterisation two or three times daily.

Erectile dysfunction

Erectile dysfunction is a common problem, occurring more often in those with diabetes than in others, and is due to neuropathy or peripheral vascular disease, or both. It is also frequently has psychogenic causes and some drugs can also be responsible. It is important that appropriate advice and treatment is sought from trained counsellors.

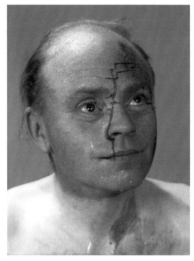

Gustatory sweating. The sweating is highlighted by starch-iodide powder

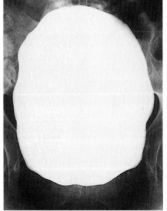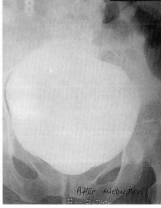

Grossly enlarged bladder before (left) and after (right) micturition

Autonomic neuropathy causes erectile impotence, which is permanent and irreversible. Retrograde ejaculation can also occur. The onset of organic impotence in neuropathy is always gradual, progressing over months or even years. Erectile ability fails first, and ejaculation declines later. Nocturnal erections are absent in these patients, whereas they are often retained in psychogenic impotence. It is often difficult to distinguish between organic and psychogenic erectile dysfunction in diabetic patients. The presence of peripheral and autonomic neuropathy makes an organic cause more likely, especially when other autonomic symptoms are present. After a full clinical examination, patients complaining of erectile dysfunction have free testosterone and serum prolactin levels measured in order to exclude other disorders, but levels are usually normal in patients with erectile dysfunction due to diabetes. There is no cure for autonomic impotence. Hormone treatment with testosterone is useless because it serves only to increase libido without improving erectile ability. In many cases, careful explanation of the cause to the affected couples will allay their fears and anxieties.

Treatment of erectile dysfunction

Diabetes centres should now offer a specialist service for advice on management of patients with erectile dysfunction. This should include psychosexual therapy which can succeed in 50% to 80% of patients who are well motivated and is also of value in conjunction with specific treatments.

Several effective specific treatments are now available: oral sildenafil is generally the first choice, and sublingual apomorphine serves as a second choice.

Oral sildenafil

This can be successful in almost two-thirds of the diabetic patients treated, which is rather less than in non-diabetic people where even higher rates of success have been reported. It is taken half to one hour before sexual activity (initial dose 50 mg; subsequently 50 to 100 mg according to response; not to be used more than once in 24 hours). Sexual stimulation and foreplay are necessary for it to be effective. It is contraindicated in those taking nitrates, those whose blood pressure is less than 90/50 mm Hg, after recent stroke or myocardial infarction, or in other situations where sexual activity is inadvisable. There are several potential side effects which are rarely troublesome (see *BNF*).

Sublingual apomorphine

This is rapidly absorbed and acts as a dopamine agonist. It is effective within 10 to 20 minutes, requiring sexual stimulation at the same time. The dose range is 2 to 3 mg. It is effective in approximately 50% of diabetic patients.

Prostaglandin preparations

Transurethral alprostadil can provide erections adequate for intercourse. An applicator for direct urethral application is provided.

Intracavernosal injection: alprostadil is now used less than previously but can be effective; modern injection systems have made its use acceptable. The side effects and contraindications are described in the *BNF*.

Vacuum devices

An external cylinder is fitted over the penis, enabling air to be pumped out, resulting in penile engorgement which is sustained by application of a ring fitted to the base of the penis. This technique is suitable for a wide range of patients and is

Features of erectile dysfunction

Organic
- Gradual onset
- Permanent
- Absent nocturnal erection
- Ejaculation often retained

Psychogenic
- Sudden onset
- Intermittent
- Nocturnal erections occur
- Penile tumescence tests give normal results

All patients complaining of erectile dysfunction should undergo a full clinical examination including examination of the external genitalia

Summary of treatments of erectile dysfunction
- Oral sildenafil
- Sublingual apomorphine
- Prostaglandin preparations
- Vacuum devices
- Penile prostheses

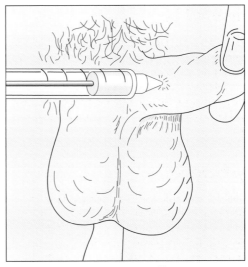

Intracavernosal injection of alprostadil

successful in most cases of erectile dysfunction, although when the problem is of long standing several attempts may be necessary before a successful erection is achieved.

Penile prostheses
Semirigid, malleable prostheses can be surgically inserted and are particularly valuable for younger patients with confirmed and permanent neuropathic impotence. Ejaculation in some patients is retained.

Diagnosis of autonomic neuropathy

Gustatory sweating is the only symptom which is almost pathognomic of diabetic autonomic neuropathy. Peripheral neuropathy (at least absent ankle jerks) must be present before the diagnosis can be made. A resting tachycardia, postural hypotension, or a gastric splash may be present.

Bedside cardiovascular tests for autonomic neuropathy are now well established: their most important role is probably in the exclusion of autonomic neuropathy. Normal and abnormal values are shown the table.

The loss of heart rate variability during deep breathing due to vagal impairment is the most reliable and simplest test of autonomic neuropathy. It is best assessed using a cardiotachograph during deep respirations (six breaths per minute) taking average readings during six breaths; it can also be performed using an ordinary electrocardiograph during a single deep breath (five seconds in, five seconds out). The heart rate difference (maximum rate during inspiration minus minimum rate during expiration) in those under 55 years old is always greater than ten. Heart rate increase on standing up should be assessed, and there should normally be an overshoot as well.

The Valsalva manoeuvre can be included among the tests: a mercury sphygmomanometer is used, the patient blowing hard into the empty barrel of a 20 ml syringe to maintain the mercury column at 40 mm Hg for 10 seconds. Maximum heart rate during blowing, followed by minimum heart rate after cessation, are recorded. There should be a bradycardia after cessation of blowing; the ratio of maximum : minimum heart rate is normally greater than 1·21 and clearly abnormal when less than 1·10. The Valsalva test should not be performed in those with proliferative retinopathy. Many other sophisticated tests need special equipment.

The figure showing the intracavernosal injection of alprostadil is from Tomlinson J, ed. *ABC of Sexual Health*. London: BMJ Publishing Group, 1999.

Normal values for autonomic function tests*

	Normal	Abnormal
Heart rate variation (deep breathing) (beats/min)	>15	<10
Increase in heart rate on standing (at 15 seconds) (beats/min)	>15	<12
Heart rate on standing 30:15 ratio	>1·04	<1·00
Valsalva ratio	>1·21	<1·20
Postural systolic pressure fall at 2 min	<10 mm Hg	>30 mm Hg

*These test results decline with age. The figures apply generally in those less than 60 years old.

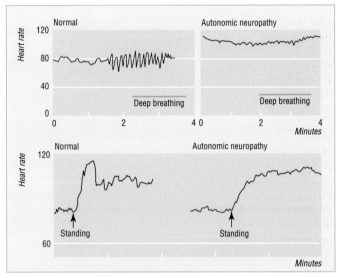

Heart rate changes in a normal subject (left) and a patient with autonomic neuropathy (right) showing loss of heart rate variation in autonomic neuropathy during deep breathing, at six breaths a minute (top), and loss of "overshoot" cardiac acceleration on standing (bottom)

14 Mononeuropathies and acute painful neuropathies

The rapid onset, severity, and eventual resolution of mononeuropathies contrast sharply with the long-term nature and irreversibility of diffuse peripheral neuropathy. The two forms of neuropathy occur quite independently of each other. Mononeuropathies are more frequently seen in Type 2 diabetic men and may even occur as the presenting symptom of diabetes.

Acute painful neuropathies

Acute painful neuropathies begin relatively acutely at any stage of diabetes, sometimes paradoxically eight to 12 weeks after starting insulin, or as the presentation of Type 2 diabetes. The acute and persistent pain can be disabling. Distribution of the pain is radicular over the territory of several adjacent nerve roots, affecting either the legs or the abdominal wall (the latter very rarely accompanied by muscle bulging from motor weakness). The thighs are affected in patients with femoral neuropathy. Both feet and legs can be affected symmetrically in a "stocking" distribution. Patients usually recover from these neuropathies in a period of six to 18 months. These neuropathies occur independently of peripheral sensory or autonomic neuropathy.

The pain causes exceptional distress because it is protracted and unremitting. Constant burning sensations, paraesthesiae or shooting pains occur, but the most characteristic symptom is a cutaneous hypersensitivity (allodynia) leading to acute discomfort on contact with clothing and bedclothes. The pain leads to insomnia and depression, and is sometimes accompanied by catastrophic weight loss. Patients are so distressed that they may seek several opinions on their condition, and often believe that they must have a malignant disease.

Treatment

This is difficult, but above all, the promise that the symptoms always eventually remit may sustain patients during the wretched months of their illness. It sometimes helps for them to meet a patient who has already recovered from neuropathic pain. Diabetic control should be optimal, and insulin should be given if necessary. Initially, simple analgesics such as paracetamol taken regularly should be tried. Tricyclic antidepressants have a specific effect in the management of neuropathic pain and are valuable in this condition: a useful combination is a preparation containing a phenothiazine (fluphenazine) with nortryptiline (Motival). Gabapentin is effective and carbamazepine may help. Capsaicin cream may have a small effect after itself causing some initial discomfort. Topiramate may be used for limited periods in those with severe and protracted pain. Drugs of addiction should be avoided although just occasionally and for a short period an opioid derivative can be used at bedtime to help distressed patients to sleep.

Application of Opsite (a thin adhesive film) can help alleviate contact discomfort. Electrical nerve stimulators applied to the site of pain may help, and patients can then take an active part in their treatment.

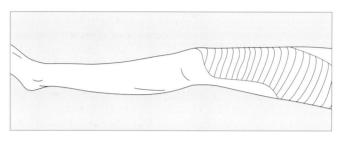
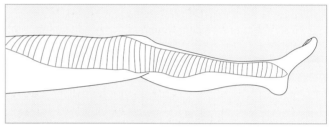

Diabetic radiculopathy area of exquisite contact sensitivity can easily and reproducibly be traced with a finger—shown in red

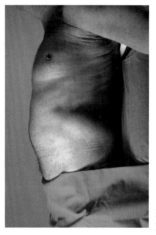

Bulging of the abdominal wall in a patient with truncal radiculopathy

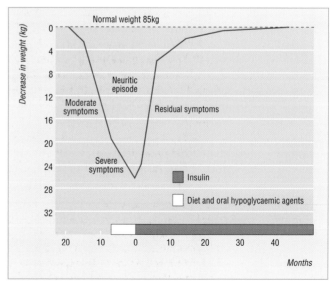

Progression of acute painful neuropathy

Femoral neuropathy

(proximal motor neuropathy or diabetic amyotrophy)

Pain with or without wasting in one or both thighs is the cardinal feature of this disagreeable condition. The quality of the pain is similar to that in painful peripheral neuropathy described above, and management is along similar lines. The knee jerk is absent while the ankle jerk is often retained. Sensation in the thigh may be altered or impaired. In some cases, motor weakness in the thigh is profound, causing falls. Other neurological disorders must be considered and excluded. Full recovery within about one year is the rule. Active physiotherapy may be needed to strengthen the wasted thigh muscles and restore mobility.

Cranial nerve palsies

Third and sixth nerve palsies presenting with diplopia of sudden onset are characteristic. Pain behind the eye occurs sometimes in third nerve palsies; the pupil is usually spared, and ptosis does not normally occur. Full examination and careful follow up are needed, but extensive investigation is not normally required. Complete recovery occurs spontaneously in about three months.

The first illustration is adapted from Bloom A, Ireland J. *A colour atlas of diabetes*, 2nd ed. London: Wolfe Publishing Ltd, 1992. The figure showing recovery from femoral neuropathy is adapted from Coppack SW, et al. *Quart J Med* 1991;79:307–13. The photograph of cranial nerve palsy is reproduced from Spillane, JD. *An atlas of clinical neurology*. Oxford: Oxford University Press.

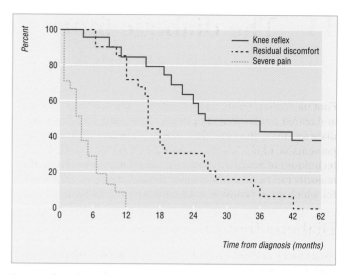

Recovery from femoral neuropathy

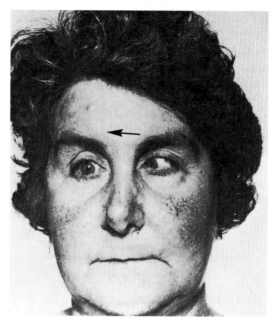

Cranial nerve palsy

15 The diabetic foot

Foot ulceration, sepsis, and amputation are universally known and feared by almost every person on hearing that they have diabetes. Yet at the same time, these are potentially the most preventable of all diabetic complications by the simplest techniques of education and care; and if lesions do occur, the majority can be cured by immediate and energetic treatment, for which good provision must be made.

Diabetic foot disorders

Neuropathy and ischaemia are the principal disorders underlying foot problems. Whenever a patient presents with an active lesion it is essential to decide at an early stage whether the foot problem is:

(a) neuropathic with an intact circulation
(b) ischaemic with (usually) or without neuropathy (neuro-ischaemic foot)
(c) critically ischaemic needing very urgent attention.

A combination of ulceration and sepsis in an ischaemic foot carries a higher risk of gangrene, and early arterial assessment and management are key to avoiding major amputation.

Men of low socioeconomic class are most prone, and Asian patients least liable, to diabetic foot disorders.

Precipitating causes of foot ulceration and infection

- Friction in ill fitting or new shoes
- Untreated callus
- Self treated callus
- Foot injuries (for example, unnoticed trauma in shoes or when walking barefoot)
- Burns (for example, excessively hot bath, hot water bottle, hot radiators, hot sand on holiday)
- Corn plaster
- Nail infections (paronychia)
- Artifactual: rarely, self-inflicted foot lesions are described and occasionally failure to heal is due to this cause
- Heel friction in patients confined to bed: it is essential that all patients confined to bed should have their heels elevated to avoid the friction which regularly causes heel blisters and sepsis, needing weeks or months of treatment, and sometimes requiring major amputation with consequent and very serious medicolegal implications.

Note: Most of the above are avoidable.

Diabetic foot problems
Neuropathic foot
• Painless
• Calluses, ulcers, sepsis, osteomyelitis
• Charcot joints, oedema, good pulses
Critically ischaemic foot
• Painful, pink, cold, no pulses

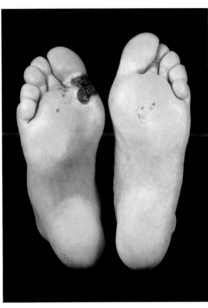

Corn plaster injury

Foot deformities predisposing to ulceration	
• Callus	• Hammer toe
• Clawed toes	• Charcot foot
• Bunions	• Deformities from previous trauma or surgery
• Pes cavus	
• Hallux rigidus	• Nail deformities
	• Oedema

Staging the diabetic foot
1 Normal
2 High risk
3 Ulcerated
4 Cellulitic
5 Necrotic
6 Major amputation

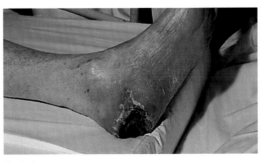

Heel ulcer

The neuropathic foot

Ulcers develop on the tips of the toes and on the plantar surfaces of the metatarsal heads and are often preceded by callus formation. If the callus is not removed then haemorrhage and tissue necrosis occur below the plaque of callus, leading to ulceration. Ulcers can be secondarily infected by staphylococci, streptococci, gram negative organisms, and anaerobic bacteria, which can quickly lead to cellulitis, abscess formation, and osteomyelitis. Sepsis complicating apical toe ulcers can lead to in situ thrombosis of the digital arteries, resulting in gangrene of the toe. The foot is invariably warm, with intact, often bounding pulses.

The ischaemic (neuro-ischaemic foot)

The absence of foot pulses must always alert physicians to the possible presence of ischaemia which requires specific assessment and often treatment as well. Lesions on the margins of the foot and absence of callus are characteristic features. Gangrene may be present as well. It is essential to identify critical ischaemia with its characteristic pink, painful (sometimes extreme and persistent pain during day and night) and pulseless, sometimes cold, foot. The ankle/brachial pressure index assessed by Doppler ultrasonography can give a useful guide to the presence or absence of ischaemia (see page 61).

Clinical features	
Neuropathic foot	**Ischaemic (neuro-ischaemic)**
• Warm with intact pulses	• Pulseless, not warm
• Diminished sensation; callus	• Usually diminished sensation
• Ulceration (usually on tips of toes and plantar surfaces under metatarsal heads)	• Ulceration (often on margins of foot, tips of toes, heels)
• Sepsis	• Sepsis
• Local necrosis	• Necrosisor gangrene
• Oedema	• Critical ischaemia (urgent attention) foot pink, painful, pulseless and often cold
• Charcot joints	

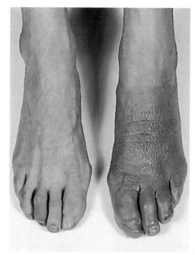

The pink, painful, ischaemic foot

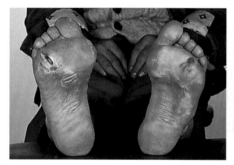

Neuropathic ulcers

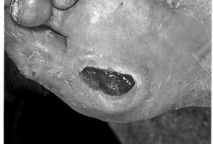

Neuropathic ulcer

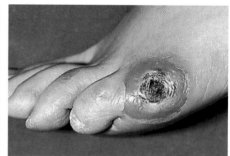

Ischaemic ulcer

Management

Infected diabetic foot lesions should be treated only by those with sufficient experience and facilities. General practitioners very rarely have such experience and should normally refer patients for specialist care.

The ulcerated foot
• Arrange urgent foot ulcer care from the specialist foot care team.
• Expect the team to ensure as a minimum:
  • local wound management, appropriate dressings, and debridement as indicated
  • antibiotic treatment as appropriate
  • investigation and management of vascular insufficiency
  • specialist footwear to distribute foot pressures appropriately
  • good blood glucose control.

Treatment of diabetic foot ulcers
Management of the ulcer falls into three parts: removal of callus, eradication of infection, and reduction of weight bearing forces, often requiring bed rest with the foot elevated. Excess keratin should be pared away with a scalpel blade by the

Six aspects of patient treatment
• Wound control
• Microbiological control
• Mechanical control
• Vascular management
• Metabolic control
• Education

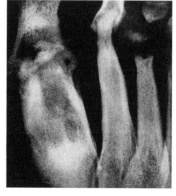

Radiograph showing osteomyelitis

podiatrist to expose the floor of the ulcer and allow efficient drainage of the lesion. A radiograph should be taken to assess the possibility of osteomyelitis whenever a deep penetrating ulcer is present, or when lesions fail to heal or continue to recur.

A bacterial swab should be taken from the floor of the ulcer after the callus has been removed; culture of excised tissue may yield even more reliable information. A superficial ulcer may be treated on an outpatient basis, and oral antibiotics prescribed according to the organisms isolated, until the ulcer has healed. The most likely organisms to infect a superficial ulcer are staphylococci, streptococci and sometimes anaerobes. Thus treatment is started with amoxycillin, flucloxacillin, and metronidazole, and adjusted when results of bacteriological culture are available. Choice and duration of antibiotic administration require considerable expertise and laboratory guidance. The patient should be instructed to carry out daily dressing of the ulcer. A simple non-adherent dressing should be applied after cleaning the ulcer with physiological saline.

Deep indolent ulcers also require local wound care and antibiotics; application of a total contact plaster cast, lightweight scotch cast boot or air cast boots which conform to the contours of the foot, thereby reducing shear forces on the plantar surface, may be used. Great care must be taken, especially with the fitting of plasters, to prevent chafing and subsequent ulcer formation elsewhere on the foot or ankle.

Any foot lesion which has not healed in one month requires further investigation and a different approach.

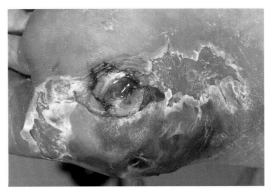
Gross sepsis leading to abscess formation

Urgent treatment

1 Bed rest.
2 Intravenous antibiotics. In the first 24 hours before bacteriological cultures are available it is necessary to provide a wide spectrum of antibiotic cover. Thus quadruple therapy may be necessary consisting of amoxycillin, flucloxacillin with metronidazole (to treat anaerobes), and either ceftazidine 1 g three times daily or gentamicin to treat gram negative organisms. This treatment can be adapted when results of bacteriological culture are available. The emergence of multiple resistant *Staphylococcus aureus* (MRSA) is presenting a very serious problem, firstly because it can be responsible for the ravages of sepsis, and secondly because these patients become "lepers", needing isolation while in hospital. Available treatments include intravenous vancomycin and intramuscular teicoplainin.
3 An intravenous insulin pump may be necessary to control the blood glucose.
4 Surgical debridement to drain pus and abscess cavities and to remove all necrotic and infected tissue including devitalised and infected bone resulting from osteomyelitis. Deep tissue swabs should be sent to the laboratory. If necrosis has developed in the digit, a ray amputation to remove the toe and part of its associated metatarsal is necessary and is usually very successful in the neuropathic foot with intact circulation. Skin grafting is occasionally needed and accelerates wound healing.

The ischaemic foot
Sepsis in the presence of ischaemia is a dangerous combination and should be treated urgently as described above. When ischaemia is suspected, or an ulcer does not respond to medical treatment, vascular investigation is required.

- Doppler studies to measure the pressure index (the ankle/brachial ratio of systolic blood pressure):
  - pressure index > 1·2 indicates rigid or calcified vessels or both
  - pressure index > 1 is normal (or calcified)

> **Danger signs: urgent treatment needed**
> - Redness and swelling of a foot which even when neuropathic causes some discomfort and pain; this clinical picture often indicates a developing abscess, and urgent surgery may be needed to save the leg
> - Cellulitis, discolouration, and crepitus (gas in soft tissues)
> - A pink, painful, pulseless foot even without gangrene indicates critical ischaemia which needs very urgent arterial investigation followed by surgical intervention whenever possible
>
> All the above require immediate hospital admission, urgent treatment, and appropriate investigation

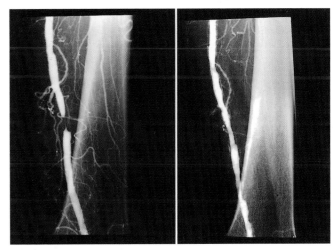
Radiograph of atheromatous narrowing of the femoral artery before and after balloon dilatation by angioplasty

- pressure index < 0·9 indicates ischaemia present
- pressure index < 0·6 indicates severe ischaemia.

   Note: Vascular calcification is common so that spuriously high readings can be obtained. This must be taken into account when the pressure index reading is evaluated.

- Arterial imaging by techniques including duplex scanning, magnetic resonance angiography, and conventional arteriography is performed with a view to angioplasty or arterial reconstruction, or both. Infrapopliteal angioplasty or distal bypass to the tibial or peroneal vessels are now well established procedures and are important for limb salvage in the diabetic foot.
- Amputation of the toe is usually unsuccessful in the neuro-ischaemic foot (in contrast to the neuropathic foot with an intact circulation) unless the foot can be revascularised. If this is not possible, then a dry necrotic toe should be allowed to autoamputate. After attempts to control infection, below knee amputation is indicated in those with rampant progressive infection or extensive tissue destruction.

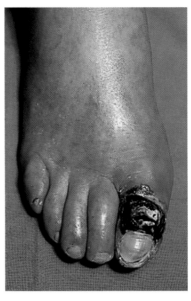

Critical ischaemia with ischaemic gangrene of great toe

   Rest pain in the severely ischaemic limb can be relieved by successful revascularisation, but if that fails, pain relief with opiates may be necessary. Paravertebral lumbar block has been disappointing in promoting healing, but occasionally rest pain is ameliorated. If all these measures fail and pain remains intractable, then below knee amputation may be needed.

Renal protection during arteriography
The intravenous dye used during angiography can precipitate acute oliguric renal failure in patients with early renal impairment. The following preventive measures should be taken:

- avoid dehydration
- give intravenous fluids starting four hours before the procedure
- intravenous insulin sliding scale should be used
- monitor urine output
- check creatinine before and on the day after the procedure.

   Note: Metformin should be stopped 48 hours before an angiographic procedure and resumed 48 hours after the procedure has been completed.

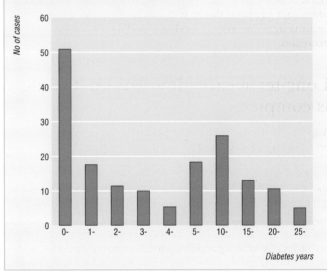

Duration of known diabetes at time of amputation

The neuropathic joint (Charcot's joint)

Loss of pain sensation together with possible rarefaction of the bones of the neuropathic foot may have serious consequences; abnormal mechanical stresses usually prevented by pain may occur, and the susceptible bones are then damaged by relatively minor trauma. Patients present with a hot swollen foot, sometimes aching, and the appearances are often mistaken for infection. Injury may have occurred days or weeks earlier, or may not even have been noticed. Sometimes Charcot changes develop after minor amputations which change the normal weight bearing stresses. Radiographs at this stage are normal, but gross damage appears and develops rapidly during the following weeks, leading to gross deformity of the foot. The destructive process does not continue indefinitely but stops after weeks or months. Bony changes are most often seen at the tarsal-metatarsal region of the foot, but they occur also at the ankle or at the metatarso-phalangeal region. Changes at other sites are rare.

   Early diagnosis is essential. The initial presentation of unilateral warmth and swelling in a neuropathic foot is extremely suggestive of a developing Charcot joint. Bone scans are more sensitive indicators of new bone formation than radiography and should be used to confirm the diagnosis. It is

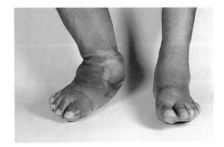

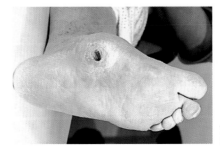

The neuropathic Charcot joint

essential to exclude infection as the cause of these changes, where the differential diagnosis can be difficult: a gallium white cell scan and a magnetic resonance imaging scan can help and are appropriate and important investigations.

Management initially comprises rest, ideally bed rest or use of non-weight bearing crutches, until the oedema and local warmth have resolved. Alternatively, the foot can be immobilised in a well moulded total contact plaster which is initially non-weight bearing. Immobilisation is continued until bony repair is complete, usually in two to three months. The use of bisphosphonates in preventing bone damage from occurring in the evolution of the Charcot foot is under investigation and appears promising. In long-term management, special shoes and insoles should be fitted to accommodate deformity and prevent ulceration, which is the major hazard of the Charcot foot.

Neuropathic oedema

Neuropathic oedema consists of swelling of the feet and lower legs associated with severe peripheral neuropathy: it is uncommon. The pathogenesis may be related to vasomotor changes and arterio-venous shunting. Ephedrine 30 mg three times daily has been shown to be useful in reducing peripheral oedema by reduction of blood flow and increase of sodium excretion.

Neuropathic oedema is associated with severe peripheral neuropathy

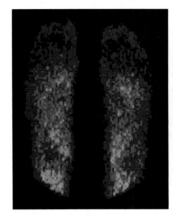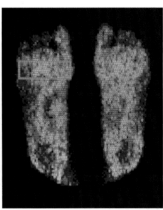

Isotope bone scans of a normal foot (left) and a neuropathic foot (right) showing high blood flow

Long-term care after wound healing is complete

Appropriate footwear, ongoing podiatry, and regular reassessment are required.

Footwear

Redistribution of weight bearing forces on vulnerable parts of the foot can be achieved by special footwear. Moulded insoles made from substances with energy absorbing properties such as plastozote and microcellular rubber are suitable for long-term redistribution of weight bearing forces. Special shoes to accommodate the shape of the foot, and moulded insoles are often necessary. In cases of severe deformity, shoes may be constructed individually for the patient. However, in most patients, extra depth "stock" shoes will usually suffice. Failure to wear appropriate shoes is commonly a cause of foot ulceration or recurrence in those who have previously had problems.

Footwear
For everyday use, especially when on your feet for long periods
- Wear a lace-up shoe, with plenty of room for the toes, and either flat or low heeled
- Do not wear slip-ons or court shoes, except for special occasions
- Do not wear slippers at home

Examination of the foot: screening and prevention

The foot must be examined routinely at the onset of diabetes and at every annual review thereafter. The key issues in assessment are listed in order of importance.

Essential
- Patient should be aware of the need for foot care.
- Identify the critically ischaemic foot.
- Active lesions should be sought (for example, hidden lesions between the toes) and treated immediately.
- Deformities, callus, skin cracks, and discoloration need to be detected and managed.
- A simple sensory test should be performed for example, a monofilament sensory test under the great toe (inability to detect 10 g or more indicates risk of foot ulceration).
- Examine the pulses (dorsalis pedis and posterior tibial).

Care and preventive measures
- Active lesions should be treated immediately
- Written advice and education on foot care should be provided
- Advice is needed on appropriate shoes to accommodate foot deformities
- Regular podiatry to remove excess callus and provide nail care is essential

Other assesments
- Assess ankle reflex.
- Assess other sensory modalities for example pinprick, vibration perception at the medial malleolus or tip of the great toe.

  Advice and education must follow the examination.

Guidelines for foot care

Low current risk foot
(normal sensation, palpable pulses)

- Individual foot care education.

At risk foot
(neuropathy, absent pulses, or other risk factor described above)

- Enhance foot care education.
- Inspect feet every three to six months.
- Advise on appropriate footwear.
- Review need for vascular assessment.
- If previous ulcer, deformity or skin changes manage as high risk.

High risk foot
(Ischaemia deformity, skin changes, or previous ulcer)

- Arrange frequent review (one to three monthly) from foot care team.
- At each review, evaluate:
  intensified foot care education
  specialist footwear and insoles
  skin and nail care according to need.
- Ensure special arrangements for people with disabilities or immobility.

The ulcerated foot
The care pathway is described on page 60.

Conclusions

Many foot problems can be prevented, and all diabetic patients should be aware of the potential problem of foot damage. Every patient should be issued with information containing straightforward safety instructions.

A good podiatrist must be available for diabetic patients. Ill-fitting shoes are the cause of many problems. New shoes should always be broken in by wearing them initially for only short periods. If the foot is in any way misshapen, for example, from bunions, hammer toes, Charcot deformities or as a result of surgery, shoes must be specially made to fit. It is a great advantage if a shoe fitter attends the chiropody clinic; it is possible to make simple shoes fit on the spot (Dru shoes for example) while awaiting delivery of more elaborate fitted shoes made in a workshop.

Close liaison between the podiatrist, orthotist, nurse, physician, and surgeon is vital in the care of the diabetic foot. The diabetic foot clinic is the optimum forum for provision of intensive podiatry, close surveillance and prompt treatment of foot infection, and the provision of specially constructed shoes.

Care of your feet
DO
- Wash feet daily with mild soap and warm water
- Check feet daily
- Seek urgent treatment for any problems
- See a podiatrist regularly
- Wear sensible shoes

DO NOT
- Use corn cures
- Use hot water bottles
- Walk barefoot
- Cut corns or callosities
- Treat foot problems yourself

Danger signs
- Check your feet every morning
- Come to the clinic *immediately* if you notice
  Swelling
  Colour change of a nail, toe, or part of a foot
  Pain or throbbing
  Breaks in the skin, including cracks, blisters, or sores

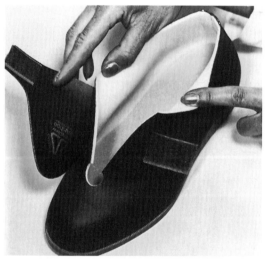

The Dru shoe

The histogram showing duration of diabetes at time of amputation adapted from Malins, J. *Clinical diabetes mellitus.* London: Eyre and Spottiswoode, 1968.

16　Diabetic nephropathy

The development of proteinuria in any diabetic patient is ominous. It is associated with a risk of severe retinopathy and neuropathy, and above all carries a major increased risk in mortality from coronary artery disease, as well as progression to renal failure in some patients. Yet developments in this field to improve the prognosis have been substantial. The overall prevalence of proteinuria in Type 1 diabetes has decreased over half a century from more than 50% of patients down to between 10 and 20%, presumably as a result of better overall diabetic care. Furthermore, at the earliest sign of proteinuria, administration of medication and very tight blood pressure control ameliorate the course of the disease and substantially delay the development of renal failure. And for those who are less fortunate, transplantation and dialysis restore a good quality of life to the majority.

Proteinuria occurs in both Type 1 diabetes and Type 2 diabetes. African-Caribbean and Asian Type 2 diabetic patients have a much higher prevalence of this disease and its associated morbidity.

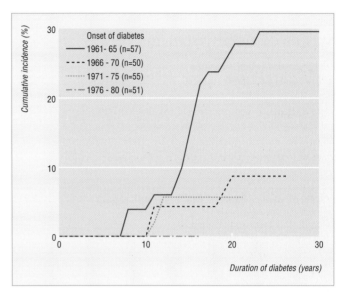

Cumulative incidence of nephropathy in patients diagnosed with Type 1 diabetes over a 20-year span

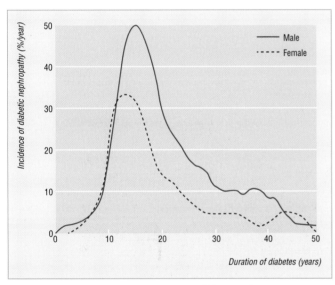

Incidence of diabetic nephropathy in Type 1 diabetic patients

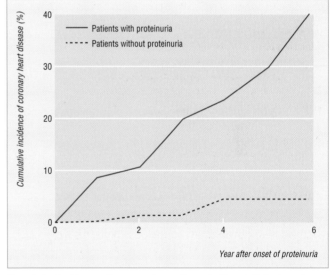

Cumulative incidence of coronary heart disease in Type 1 diabetic patients with and without proteinuria

Onset of nephropathy

The earliest detectable development in Type 1 diabetes of small amounts of proteinuria (microalbuminuria) occurs more than five years after diagnosis. Both micro and gross albuminuria are detected at diagnosis in many with Type 2 diabetes, both because diabetes may already be long standing and in some instances because of established hypertension or other renal diseases.

Initiating factors and progression promoters in diabetic nephropathy

Factors leading to initiation and those determining rate of progression of diabetic renal disease are gaining increasing recognition.

Both development and early progression of diabetic nephropathy are most likely to occur following years of poor

Nephropathy—initiating factors and progression promoters

Initiating factors	Progression promoters
• Persistently poor diabetic control	• Blood pressure
• Hypertension in Type 2 diabetes	• Proteinuria
• Genetic factors	• Persistently poor diabetic control
	• Dyslipidaemia
	• Genetic factors
	• Smaller kidneys (or glomeruli)
	• Smoking
	• High dietary protein

diabetic control; tight control over a decade both delays onset of the disease and slows progression chiefly of its early phase, although there is some effect in established disease as well. There is also a familial propensity to nephropathy in both Type 1 and Type 2 diabetes, although the precise genetic factors responsible have not been identified.

Stages of nephropathy

Early physiological changes

At the onset of Type 1 diabetes there is evidence of hyperfiltration with increased glomerular filtration rate, and large kidneys and glomeruli. These defects can be reversed by meticulous diabetic control; there is however no good evidence that these changes predispose to the subsequent development of nephropathy.

> **The most powerful factor in slowing progression of the disease is the skilful and timely use of angiotensin converting enzyme (ACE) inhibitors and angiotensin receptor blockers, together with the strict management of hypertension when it occurs**

Stages of progression of diabetic nephropathy

	Normal (I)	Incipient (II)	Persistent (III)	Clinical (IV)	End stage (V)
Albuminuria (mg/24 h)	<20	20–300 (microalbuminuria)	≥300 (up to 15 g/day)	≥300 (up to 15 g/day)	≥300 (can fall)
Glomerular filtration rate (ml/min)	High/normal Hyperfiltration	Normal/high	Normal or decreased	Decreased	Greatly decreased
Serum creatinine (μmol/l)	Normal 60-100	Normal 60-120	High normal 80-120	High 120-400	Very high >400
Blood pressure (mm Hg)	Normal	Slightly increased	Increased	Increased	Increased
Clinical signs	None	None	Anaemia ± oedema, increased blood pressure, may be none	Anaemia ± oedema, increased blood pressure, may be none	Anaemia oedema, increased blood pressure, uraemic symptoms

Course of nephropathy

The natural course of diabetic nephropathy is the progression through five stages from normal renal function to end-stage renal failure as shown in the table. Incipient nephropathy, identified by the appearance of microalbuminuria, is the earliest clinical stage and is not associated with significant clinical signs or any changes other than a very small increase in blood pressure. At this stage urine testing by conventional methods will give negative or only trace positive results.

As the disease progresses albuminuria increases until end-stage nephropathy, when it may decrease; there are wide variations in the amount of protein excretion. The glomerular filtration rate shows a progressive decline, which varies considerably between patients and is usefully assessed by calculating the inverse creatinine value (1/serum creatinine concentration) which can be plotted against time and is generally linear. Blood pressure rises progressively. The nephropathy is commonly asymptomatic until it is advanced, when oedema and breathlessness develop. Anaemia often occurs relatively early in the course of the disease before renal failure is established, and much sooner than in non-diabetic renal disease, as a result of diminished erythropoietin production, which can be corrected by injections of erythropoietin, sometimes with considerable clinical benefit.

Hyperlipidaemia is common in nephropathy, as are other risk factors for vascular disease, including changes in the concentrations of fibrinogen and other clotting factors.

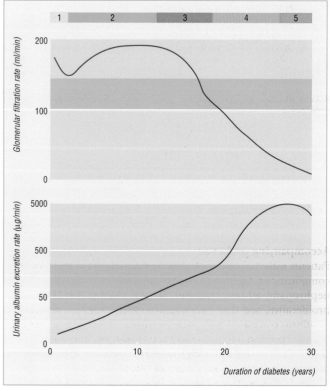

Natural history of diabetic nephropathy in Type 1 diabetes

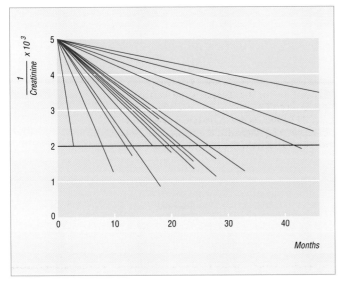

Decline of renal function in 16 Type 1 diabetic patients with nephropathy

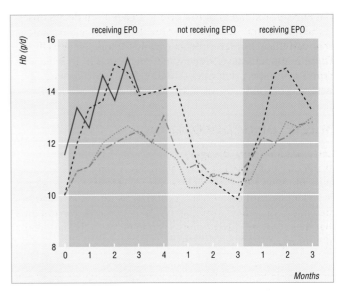

Erythropoietin (EPO) deficient anaemia in early diabetic nephropathy treated successfully with EPO injections

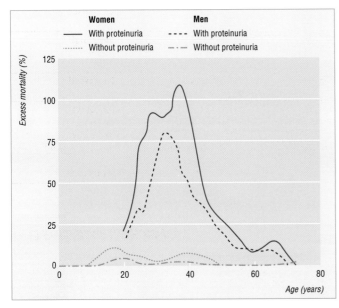

Relative mortality of Type 1 diabetic patients with and without persistent proteinuria

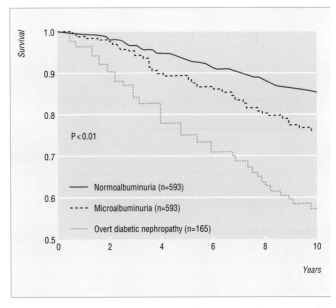

Survival curves of Type 1 diabetic patients with respect to all cause mortality in relation to presence or absence of proteinuria

Accompanying problems

Patients with diabetic nephropathy normally have many other complications, the problems increasing as the stage of nephropathy advances. Almost all have retinopathy, often proliferative, and they have a tenfold increased risk of blindness compared with patients without proteinuria. A very high proportion have coronary artery disease, with an excess risk of death many times higher than in patients without proteinuria. They are also more at risk of peripheral vascular disease (often with vascular calcification, peripheral and autonomic neuropathy, foot ulceration, and amputation.

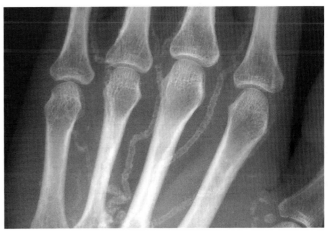

Radiograph of a hand showing extensive vascular calcification

Primary prevention

Poor diabetic control predisposes to the development of nephropathy, although it is not the only factor, and genetic components also predispose to this disease. Tight control of diabetes early in its course helps to delay development of nephropathy (see chapter 10). Many patients will never acquire proteinuria even after several decades. Blood pressure management at all stages is crucial (see below).

Early detection and diagnosis

Testing urine samples for the presence of protein or microalbuminuria should be routine practice at every clinic visit and is obligatory at the annual review. If proteinuria develops it is important to distinguish the onset of nephropathy from other causes of renal disease.

Microalbuminuria is detected by measurement of the albumin/creatinine ratio or urinary albumin concentration. The test is best performed on the first morning urine sample. If albuminuria is discovered for the first time, confirmation is required within one month if proteinuria is present, and if microalbuminuria is detected it should be confirmed twice within the ensuing months. All laboratory and near patient commercial tests specifically designed for microalbuminuria have satisfactory sensitivity (>80%) and specificity (>90%).

If proteinuria has evolved gradually over several years in the presence of retinopathy, and there are no unusual features such as haematuria, unequal size kidneys, or a history of urinary tract complaints, then extensive investigation is not necessary. In Type 2 diabetes, however, there is a greater chance of non-diabetic renal disease being present, and renal biopsy may be needed, especially if there are atypical features. In both Type 1 diabetes and Type 2 diabetes the absence of retinopathy should make one suspect other causes of renal failure. Indeed, rapid onset of proteinuria in any patient is never due to diabetes and should always be fully investigated, including a biopsy.

The characteristic pathological lesion is diabetic glomerulosclerosis, including basement membrane thickening, mesangial expansion, and in the later stages, the classical Kimmelstiel-Wilson nodules, together with hyalinisation of efferent and afferent arterioles. Mesangial expansion, which requires an experienced pathologist to interpret, correlates well with renal function.

Management

- Tight diabetic control delays the onset and slows the progression chiefly in the early phase of the disease, with a smaller effect in fully established disease.
- Established microalbuminuria (—that is three positive samples) is managed with ACE inhibitors:
  (a) in Type 1 diabetes treatment is commenced regardless of blood pressure which should in any case be maintained < 130/80 mm Hg, or 125/75 mm Hg, in younger patients
  (b) in Type 2 diabetes treatment aims to maintain a blood pressure < 130/80 mm Hg.

  ACE inhibitors and angiotensin receptor blockers always reduce microalbuminuria and delay the onset of established proteinuria.

- Established proteinuria (proteinuria > 500 mg/24 h or albuminuria > 300 mg/24 h).

Diagnostic categories

Microalbuminuria
- Albumin creatinine ratio >2·5 mg/mmol/l (men) >3·5 mg/mmol/l (women)
- Urinary albumin concentration >20 mg/l
- Urinary albumin excretion rate 30-300 mg/24 h, or 20-200 µg/min in an overnight specimen

Proteinuria
- Urinary albumin excretion rate >300 mg/24 h
- Urinary protein excretion >500 mg/24 h (albumin creatinine ration >30 mg/min; albumin concentration >200 mg/l)

Investigations in a patient with proteinuria

- Midstream urine
- 24 hour urine protein
- Renal ultrasonography
- Blood count
- Erythrocyte sedimentation rate
- Antinuclear factor
- Serum complement
- Serum lipids
- (Renal biopsy only as indicated)

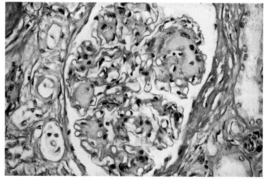

Diabetic glomerulosclerosis showing Kimmelstiel-Wilson nodules

This phase is always managed by vigorous hypotensive treatment now aiming where possible for a blood pressure of < 130/80 mm Hg or even less (125/75 mm Hg) in younger patients. This both reduces (or occasionally eliminates) proteinuria and slows progression of the declining glomerular filtration rate, best demonstrated in Type 1 diabetes, and is also protective in some aspects of cardiovascular disease (see below).

- Dyslipidaemia. Detection and management of hyperlipidaemias is important because of the huge increase in cardiovascular disease in those with nephropathy. The idea, however, that reducing lipidaemia slows the progression of the renal disease is unproven.
- Restricting protein intake has a small beneficial effect on the decline in glomerular filtration rate but unless the intake is very high (greater than 1 g/kg/day) restriction is not normally advised.
- Oral hypoglycaemic treatment in Type 2 diabetes must be reviewed: metformin should not be used when renal function is impaired because of the danger of lactic acidosis; also long acting, renally excreted sulphonylureas, notably glibenclamide, should not be used because of the risk of accumulation and hypoglycaemia. Drugs such as gliclazide which are mainly metabolised are preferable (see page 15).
- Anaemia often occurs relatively early in the course of the disease before renal failure is established, and much sooner than in non-diabetic renal disease, as a result of diminished erythropoietin production, which can be corrected by injections of erythropoietin, sometimes with considerable clinical benefit.
- Smoking should be strongly discouraged.
- Regular reassessment and management of all the other diabetic complications to which diabetic nephropathy patients are especially prone is extremely important in those who develop this disease.

Choice of antihypertensive agent

ACE inhibitors or angiotensin receptor blockers are the agents of choice for diabetic nephropathy patients at any stage. They probably provide benefits over and above their blood pressure lowering effects in comparison with other agents. However, the overriding need is to maintain good blood pressure control in all those with nephropathy using any hypotensive agent to suit the individual patient, and indeed for Type 2 diabetes, United Kingdom Prospective Diabetes Study (UKPDS) demonstrated no drug preferential benefit. Combinations of drugs are almost always required, especially in overweight Type 2 diabetic individuals when more than two drugs are often needed: the ideal blood pressure of <130/80 mm Hg may be difficult to achieve and some compromise following informed discussion with patients may be necessary. Tight blood pressure control may induce or exacerbate postural hypotension, which should be avoided.

For microalbuminuria

Even in normotensive patients, aim to titrate medication to reduce or eliminate microalbuminuria. Doses often needed are:
- ACE inhibitors*: enalapril 10 mg twice daily
  lisinopril 20 mg daily
  ramipril 2·5 mg daily.
- Angiotensin 2 receptor antagonists*†:
  irbesartan 300 mg daily
  losartan 50 mg daily.

*Only some of the longest established and therefore most studied agents are mentioned here by name. Many others are available and can be found in the *BNF*.
†Angiotensin 2 antagonists do not cause the cough often induced by ACE inhibitors, but are more expensive than the latter.

Treatment of nephropathy
- Optimal diabetic control
- Antihypertensive treatment and diuretics
- Reduce hyperlipidaemia
- Stop smoking

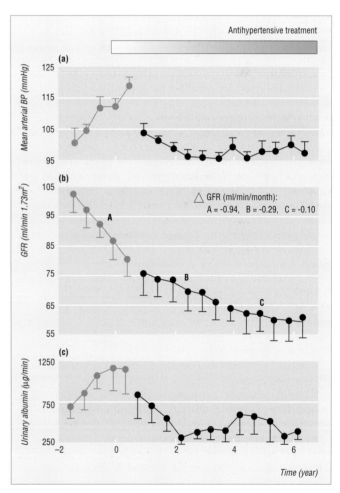

Antihypertensive treatment reduces the decline of glomerular filtration rate (GFR) in patients with Type 1 diabetes

For hypertension
ACE inhibitors (or angiotensin 2 antagonists) to which may be added:

- calcium channel blockers (amlodipine)
- diuretics
- β blockers
- others.

For African-Caribbeans a calcium channel blocker such as verapamil may be a first choice hypotensive agent.

Creatinine should always be checked within one to two weeks of starting treatment with a ACE inhibitor or angiotensin 2 antagonist in case a rapid rise occurs in patients with renal artery stenosis. In this case, the patient should be changed to another agent, and appropriate investigations undertaken as well. For further information on treatment of hypertension, specific indications and contraindications to individual drugs, see chapter 17.

Patient counselling
Considerable fear is generated when patients are told that they have "kidney damage", with visions of dialysis and transplantation. This is needlessly and carelessly damaging to patient well being; the proper context of the disease must be presented by physicians and nurse educators.

Renal failure
Patients with end-stage renal failure need much time and consideration. Renal support therapy is now available for most of these patients, who should be assessed by a nephrologist once the serum creatinine exceeds 150 μmol/l. Transplantation or dialysis is often necessary at a lower serum creatinine concentration than in non-diabetic people, often around 450 to 550 μmol/l. Kidney transplantation is the treatment of choice if the patient has good cardiac function, and cardiac and peripheral vascular assessments are essential before treatment becomes necessary. Results of renal transplantation are shown in the table. If cardiac function is severely compromised them continuous ambulatory peritoneal dialysis (CAPD) is preferable as long-term treatment. Long-term haemodialysis is used chiefly for those who cannot cope with CAPD for reasons of blindness, lack of manual dexterity or intellectual decline. One year after starting CAPD more than 70% of patients are alive, and even after five years approximately 40% survive.

Pancreas transplantation
Combined kidney and pancreas transplantation is undertaken at some major centres and aims to eliminate diabetes and with it the need for insulin injections. Patients who are liberated from decades of restrictions and self discipline imposed by diabetes experience a joy and happiness rarely witnessed in medical practice. This is the prime reason for offering combined transplantation. Other benefits derive from slowing the redevelopment of glomerulosclerosis in the transplanted kidney, and halting the progression of neuropathy. Retinopathy which by this stage has almost always been laser treated is unaffected. The future potential for islet cell transplantation is briefly described on page 22.

Management of diabetes during transplantation and dialysis

At transplantation
Continuous intravenous insulin infusion is always used; soluble insulin diluted in physiological saline at 1 unit/ml. Infusion

---

Counselling for patients with nephropathy

Physicians and nurse educators should explain that:

- Not all of those (approximately 20%) with microalbuminuria will go on to develop established nephropathy
- Many of those with microalbuminuria or even established nephropathy will not progress to end-stage renal failure
- Modern treatment properly taken is highly effective in retarding disease progression

---

Approximate expected survival after cadaver renal transplantation

	1 year	5 years
Patient survival (diabetic/non-diabetic)	90/95%	80/88%
Graft survival* (diabetic/non-diabetic)	75/85%	55/75%

*Graft survival includes death with a functioning graft

Approximate expected survival rates after pancreas and renal transplantation

	1 year	5 years
Patient survival (diabetic)	95%	80%
Functioning pancreas graft survival	85%	60%
Functioning kidney graft survival	90%	70%

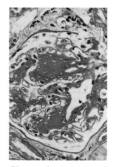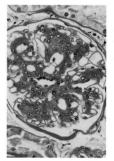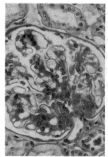

Glomerulus showing changes of diabetic glomerulosclerosis (left) followed by illustrations at five years (middle) and 10 years (right) after pancreatic transplant, showing considerable resolution after 10 years

rates vary considerably, usually in the range 2 to 20 units/h; during high dose steroid treatment the higher infusion rates are often needed. Intravenous insulin infusion is continued until drips have been taken down and the patient can eat: the insulin regimen to be followed thereafter is described in chapter 9. The daily dose is started about 20% above the pre-transplant dose and adjustments thereafter are made by trial and error.

During peritoneal dialysis

With solutions of low glucose content (1·36% glucose) no adjustment to the normal insulin regimen is needed. Dialysates of high glucose content can however severely disrupt diabetes and additional insulin is needed. During CAPD insulin can be administered entirely from the dialysis bags: soluble insulin is added to each bag, initially using the existing total daily dose in divided amounts, often giving less at night. The dose may eventually be quite different from that given subcutaneously. The technique is often satisfactory and excellent control can be achieved without hypoglycaemia. Patients whose technique is poor, and who are thus liable to peritonitis, should not be given intra-peritoneal insulin. The use of dialysis fluids with high glucose content (3·86%), needed to alleviate fluid overload, causes havoc with diabetes control; additional soluble insulin (in a dose appropriately titrated) must be given before administration of the strong glucose concentrations, or possibly more effectively, additional insulin given intra-peritoneally.

Rejection

High doses of steroids always upset diabetes within a few hours. This problem may be anticipated by increasing the first insulin dose after steroids have been given. Intravenous insulin infusion (about 4 units/h) for a few hours as a supplement to the normal subcutaneous insulin is almost always needed until the administration of methylprednisolone has been completed.

Non-diabetic renal disease

Some patients, especially those with Type 2 diabetes, develop unrelated non-diabetic renal disorders. Clues to their presence have been presented above, but renal artery stenosis should be particularly mentioned. This is most common in Type 2 diabetic patients with hypertension and peripheral vascular disease. Full renal assessment including ultrasound examination is essential, although renal arteriography is often required to confirm or exclude the diagnosis. The distinction is vital as ACE inhibitors may provoke considerable deterioration in renal function or even precipitate renal failure.

Urinary tract infections

Urinary tract infections occur in diabetic people with the same frequency as in those without diabetes, but they are sometimes exceptionally severe and may cause the renal papillae to slough, causing necrotising papillitis, or rarely emphysematous cystitis with air in the bladder wall. Infection is particularly troublesome in the rare patient with urinary retention from neurogenic bladder. Diabetic control is easily disturbed by urinary infection, as with any infection, and must be regained quickly, with insulin if necessary, while the infection is treated with antibiotics.

Pyelonephritis with septicaemia is not uncommon in diabetes, with occasional formation of a perinephric abscess. The source of the infection may not be immediately apparent and sometimes patients present in profound shock without an obvious site of infection.

Renal protection during arteriography

The intravenous dye used during angiography can precipitate acute oliguric renal failure in patients with early renal impairment. The following preventive measures should be taken:

- Avoid dehydration
- Give intravenous fluids starting four hours before the procedure
- Intravenous insulin sliding scale should be used
- Monitor urine output
- Check creatinine before and on the day after the procedure

Note: Metformin should be stopped 48 hours before an angiographic procedure and resumed 48 hours after the procedure has been completed

---

Glomerulonephritis and other renal disorders can occur in diabetic patients and require renal biopsy for diagnosis and treatment in their own right

---

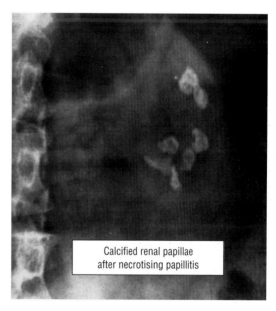

Calcified renal papillae
after necrotising papillitis

Radiograph showing calcified renal papillae after necrotising papillitis

The figure showing incidence of diabetic nephropathy is adapted from Anderson, AR. *Diabetologia* 1983;25:496–501. Cumulative incidence of nephropathy in patients diagnosed with diabetes over a 20-year span is adapted from Bojestig M, et al. *New Engl J Med* 1994;330:15-18. The cumulative incidence of coronary heart disease is adapted from Jensen T, et al. *Diabetologia* 1987;30:114-18. The graph showing treatment with erythropoietin is adapted from Watkins, P. *Diab Med* 1999;16:1-7. The figure showing relative mortality of diabetic patients with and without persistent proteinuria is adapted from Borck-Johnsson K, et al. *Diabetologia* 1985;28:590-6. The figure showing survival curves with respect to all cause mortality is adapted from Rossing P, et al. *BMJ* 1996;313:779-84. The figure showing antihypertensive treatment reduces the decline of glomerular filtration rate in patients with Type 1 diabetes is adapted from Parving H-H, et al. *BMJ* 1987;294:1443-7. The slide of glomerulus showing changes of diabetic glomerulosclerosis is reproduced from Fioretto P, et al. *New Engl J Med* 1998;339:69-75. Copyright Massachussetts Medical Society.

17 Cardiovascular disease, hypertension, lipids, and myocardial infarction

Diabetic patients, particularly those with Type 2 diabetes and those with proteinuria, are at very considerable risk of excessive morbidity and mortality from cardiovascular, cerebrovascular and peripheral vascular disease leading to myocardial infarction (MI), strokes and amputations. Much effort must be given to reducing as far as possible the risk factors which are known to predispose to major atheromatous arterial disease. Many effective measures can now be taken, adding considerably to the complexity of treating diabetic patients, especially those with Type 2 diabetes. The difficulties and dangers of polypharmacy are discussed on page 14.

> *The glycaemic disturbance (of Type 2 diabetes) may be mild, but the rest of the disease is not*
> **George Alberti, 1988**

Coronary artery disease

Cardiovascular disease is substantially increased in diabetes, hyperglycaemia representing an independent risk factor. It is the chief cause of death and this observation strongly influences the management of diabetes by the important focus on reducing the risk factors responsible.

Diabetes more than doubles the risk of cardiovascular disease. In the United Kingdom, 35% of deaths are attributable to cardiovascular causes, compared with about 60% in those with Type 2 diabetes, and 67% of Type 1 diabetic patients alive after 40 years of age. The relative risk is greater for women than for men, so that the sex ratio is equal in those with diabetes, with a loss of the usual male predominance. The development of MI over a period of seven years in middle-aged diabetic patients without known pre-existing coronary heart disease (CHD) is the same as that in non-diabetics with existing CHD. The presence of proteinuria and even microalbuminuria is associated with a particularly large risk of CHD and a high mortality from MI
(see page 65).

Those at especially high risk of developing CHD include

- Smokers
- Hypertensives
- Those with insulin resistance associated with obesity
- Patients of Asian origin
- Those with microalbuminuria
- Those with diabetic nephropathy (macroalbuminuria)
- Those with poor glycaemic control (16% increased risk of MI for every 1% increase in HbA_{1c})
- Those with hyperlipidaemic states

Prevention of cardiovascular disease: effects of lowering blood pressure
Those with a high risk of cardiovascular disease stand to gain proportionately greater benefit by reduction of risk factors. Two recently published major trials demonstrated exactly what can be achieved.

The United Kingdom Prospective Diabetes Study (UKPDS; published in 1998, see page 42): tight *v* less tight blood pressure control (mean 144/82 mm Hg *v* 154/87 mm Hg). Benefits:

- heart failure reduced by 56%
- strokes reduced by 44%
- combined MI, sudden death, stroke, peripheral vascular disease reduced by 34% (MI alone was reduced non-significantly by 16%).

There were also considerable benefits on the development of retinopathy and proteinuria (see page 43).

Heart Outcomes Prevention Evaluation (HOPE) and MicroHOPE study: this study over 4·5 years comprised 9297 patients overall and included 3577 diabetic patients (98% with Type 2 diabetes). Patients with diabetes and one other risk factor for cardiovascular disease were randomly treated with the

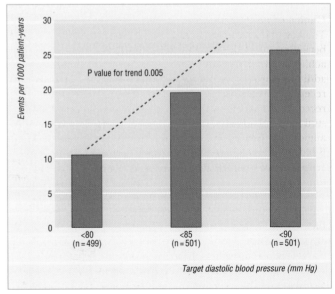

Rates of serious cardiovascular events according to target diastolic blood pressure in 1500 patients with hypertension and Type 2 diabetes

angiotensin converting enzyme (ACE) inhibitor ramipril 10 mg daily or placebo. Systolic blood pressure decreased by approximately 2 to 3 mm Hg and yielded a reduction of combined MI, strokes, and deaths from cardiovascular diseases of 25%.

The demonstrated benefits included:

- MI relative risk reduced by 22%
- stroke relative risk reduced by 33%
- cardiovascular death relative risk reduced by 37%.

It was concluded that ACE inhibitors were the first line treatment for blood pressure control in diabetes. Despite some caveats relating to the handling of the study, this treatment should probably be extended to normotensive patients with high cardiovascular risks.

There have been several other published multicentre trials: the results of the HOPE and other studies are well summarised by Bilous R, HOPE and other recent trials of antihypertensive therapy in Type 2 diabetes; in Amiel S ed. *Horizons in Medicine*, Royal College of Physicians of London, 2002.

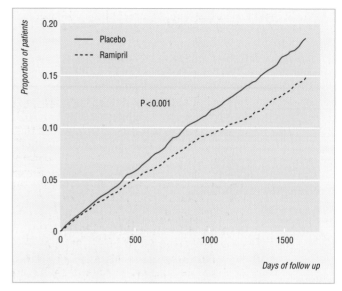

Kaplan-Meier estimates of the composite outcome of myocardial infarction, stroke, or death from cardiovascular causes in the ramipril group and the placebo group in the HOPE study

Blood pressure management

Blood pressure should be checked annually or more frequently as indicated. Borderline readings should be re-checked several times before the decision to use medication is taken. Before using pharmacological agents, the measures shown in the box all have some effect on reducing blood pressure:

Blood pressure > 160/100 mm Hg should always be treated in those with and without diabetes aiming for a level of <140/80 mm Hg (audit standard <140/90 mm Hg).

Blood pressure 140-159/90-99 mm Hg should be treated in diabetic patients, most aggressively in those with cardiovascular risk factors, especially if there is evidence of end organ damage; aim for <140/80 mm Hg.

Blood pressure > 140/80 mm Hg should be treated if there is evidence of target organ damage or if the 10-year CHD risk exceeds 15%, aiming for a level <140/80 mm Hg. Blood pressure >130/80 mm Hg should be treated in those with microalbuminuria or macroalbuminuria (see page 68).

Choice of antihypertensive drugs

The key objective is to lower blood pressure by any means because most of the benefits relate to the blood pressure achieved rather than the drug used. There are however additional advantages using ACE inhibitors or angiotensin 2 receptor antagonists (see page 68). Indeed, results of the recent losartan intervention for end point reduction (LIFE) study showed additional benefits resulting from the use of the angiotensin 2 receptor antagonist losartan when compared with β blocker atenolol, despite comparable blood pressure reduction. Many, probably most, patients will need more than one drug to achieve the intended goal. A pragmatic approach to treatment it is often needed.

ACE inhibitors or angiotensin 2 receptor blockers are the first choice in those with microalbuminuria. ACE inhibitors, angiotensin 2 receptor blockers, cardioselective β blockers or thiazide diuretics are reasonable first line treatment in those without microalbuminuria. Long acting dihydropyridine calcium channel antagonists (for example, amlodipine) have an important role in treating hypertension and are second line agents.

Factors that affect blood pressure

- Salt restriction
- Weight reduction or exercise programmes
- Reduction of excessive alcohol intake

First and foremost, the key objective when choosing antihypertensive drugs is to lower blood pressure by any means because most of the benefits relate to the blood pressure achieved rather than the drug used

Guidelines for choice of antihypertensive drugs

- Those with heart failure should have an ACE inhibitor whenever possible, which can be combined with a diuretic
- Conversion to an angiotensin 2 receptor blocker is helpful if a patient develops cough on an ACE inhibitor
- Addition of an angiotensin 2 receptor blocker to an ACE inhibitor will have an additive benefits on blood pressure but not on microalbuminuria
- Blood pressure in some African and Caribbean patients may respond better to calcium channel antagonists and diuretics than to other agents

Lipids and diabetes

Hyperlipidaemias also commonly exist in those with diabetes and increase still further the risk of ischaemic heart disease, especially in Type 2 diabetes. Detection and control of hyperlipidaemia can effectively reduce MI, coronary deaths and overall mortality. Indeed, even when low density lipoprotein (LDL) cholesterol is normal or even slightly raised in Type 2 diabetes (the major abnormalities being low HDL cholesterol and high triglyceride) the LDL particles may be qualitatively different and more atherogenic.

Screening for dyslipidaemia
This is an essential aspect of the annual review. If the lipid profile is entirely normal, further screening could be postponed for three to five years unless circumstances change. An elevated triglyceride needs confirmation when fasting.

Diabetic control
Optimising diabetic control often improves an abnormal lipid profile in Type 1 diabetes and sometimes in Type 2 diabetes.

Other medications and alcohol
Some drugs and also a high alcohol intake disturb plasma lipids (see table) and this aspect of treatment must be examined and if necessary modified.

Lifestyle measures
The importance of stopping smoking, weight reduction and exercise are described in chapter 3. Advice on low fat diets is also needed. Hypertension must be treated.

Lipid modifying drugs
Statins are the first line of drugs for treating hypercholesterolaemia; and fibrates for treating hypertriglyceridaemia. Statins and fibrates can be used alone or together for treating mixed hyperlipidaemia. Specialist advice should be taken on resistant or complex hyperlipidaemic states.

Targets for treatment
The current targets for cholesterol and other lipid fractions are now the same for primary prevention in diabetes as for secondary prevention in people without diabetes. They are as follows:

- total cholesterol <5·0 mmol/l
- fasting triglyceride <2·0 mmol/l
- LDL cholesterol <3·0 mmol/l
- high density lipoprotein (HDL) cholesterol >1·1 mmol/l.

It is desirable that the ratio (HDL cholesterol)/(total cholesterol − HDL cholesterol) should be >0·25. Alternatively, the total cholesterol/HDL cholesterol should be <3.0.

There is much debate as to whether lipid lowering agents are of any value if started over the age of 75 years.

Heart Protection Study
This huge double blind trial of 20 000 people at increased risk of vascular disease examined the benefits of treatment with simvastatin 40 mg daily, and reported its results in March 2002 (see further reading list). The vascular event rate curves began to separate by the end of the first year, and the absolute benefits of treatment were seen to increase over time, becoming very obvious after five to six years. The major results are shown overleaf.

Some causes of secondary hyperlipidaemia

	Main lipid abnormalities
Alcohol abuse	↑ Triglyceride, ↑ HDL
Therapeutic drugs (diuretics, oral contraceptives retinoids, corticosteroids, anabolic steroids, progestogens related to testosterone)	↑ Triglyceride or cholesterol or both, ↓ HDL
Hypothyroidism	↑ Cholesterol
Chronic renal failure	↑ Triglyceride
Nephrotic syndrome	↑ Cholesterol, ± ↑ triglyceride
Cholestasis	↑ Cholesterol
Bulimia	↑ Triglyceride
Anorexia nervosa	↑ Cholesterol
Pregnancy	↑ Triglyceride

Targets for blood lipids control suggested by the European Diabetes Policy Group

	Low risk	At risk	High risk
Serum total cholesterol			
mmol/l	<4·8	4·8-6·0	>6·0
mg/dl	<185	184-230	>230
Serum LDL cholesterol			
mmol/l	<3·0	3·0-4·0	>4·0
mg/dl	<115	115-155	>155
Serum HDL cholesterol			
mmol/l	>1·2	1·0-1·2	<1·0
mg/dl	>46	39-46	<39
Serum triglycerides			
mmol/l	<1·7	1·7-2·2	>2·2
mg/dl	<150	150-200	>200

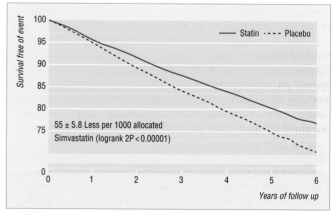

Simvastatin: vascular event by follow up duration

- reduction in vascular deaths   17%
- reduction in major vascular events   24%
- reduction in strokes   27%.

Treatment benefits were not only obvious among patients who had previously had an MI but also in those with prior cerebrovascular or peripheral vascular disease. Benefits were also demonstrated for diabetic patients without previous CHD. Both sexes benefited equally, and elderly patients over 75 years of age were seen to benefit to the same extent as younger patients.

The implications of the results of this study for diabetic patients are obvious, and serious consideration with regard to offering treatment with a statin drug must be given.

Severe hyperlipidaemic states

Extreme mixed hyperlipidaemias are, on rare occasions, associated with uncontrolled diabetes. The plasma has a milky appearance, and xanthomata appear in the skin as bright yellow papules particularly at the elbows, knees and buttocks. Even the retina assumes the pallor of lipaemia retinalis described as the "peaches and cream" appearance. The condition normally resolves when glycaemic control is achieved, lipid levels often return to normal, and the xanthomata disappear. Most but not all patients have Type 2 diabetes. The condition needs to be carefully monitored, and it is often wise to administer lipid lowering drugs until resolution. Sometimes they need to be continued indefinitely.

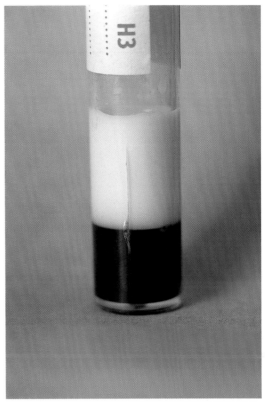

Milky plasma of severe hyperlipidiaemia

Myocardial infarction (MI)

The greater risk of CHD in diabetic patients is accompanied by a greater risk of MI: approximately 10% of all MIs occur in diabetic patients. Unfortunately, mortality rates are also about twofold higher. The increased mortality is attributable to left ventricular dysfunction leading to left ventricular failure and cardiogenic shock.

Presentation of MI in those with diabetes is the same as in those without, although a greater proportion lack chest pain. Absence of cardiac pain has been attributed to the cardiac denervation although this concept lacks conviction.

Treatment

Thrombolysis
This should be used in diabetic patients for the same indications as for non-diabetics. The risk of vitreous haemorrhage in those with proliferative retinopathy is negligible. The benefits to diabetic patients with MI appears even greater than to those without diabetes.

Aspirin 300 mg
Given at the onset of a MI, enteric coated aspirin 75-150 mg daily should be continued indefinitely thereafter.

Insulin treatment
Commenced at the onset of an MI, insulin treatment leading to optimal glycaemic control confers benefits on reducing mortality after discharge from hospital. The DIGAMI (Diabetes, Insulin, Glucose infusion in Acute Myocardial Infarction) study examined 620 patients with established or newly diagnosed diabetes (plasma glucose exceeding 11·1 mmol/l): an insulin and glucose infusion was started at presentation, followed by a multiple insulin injection regimen for at least three months. Twelve-month mortality was reduced by 30%. Confirmation of these results is required, but at present this study presents the best evidence available for the management of diabetes after MI.

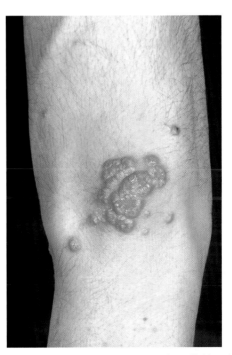

Xanthomata on the knee from severe hyperlipidaemia

All diabetic patients, newly diagnosed and with established disease should be treated with insulin, and in many, this should be continued indefinitely. Some discretion needs to be used among elderly patients, or others who cannot easily or comfortably use insulin, in whom other simple measures can also achieve very good diabetic control.

Coronary artery bypass grafts and angioplasty

Decisions advising on the need for invasive coronary artery treatments are made in the same way as for non-diabetics. Coronary artery bypass grafts may offer an improved prognosis to those with diabetes after spontaneous Q wave infarction compared with angioplasty, and further investigations of this apparent benefit are in progress.

After MI

Half the patients after their first MI die during the following twelve months, and half of those die before they reach hospital. Continuing optimal management of all risk factors is strongly recommended.

Management of risk factors after MI

- Cessation of smoking
- Optimal blood pressure management
- Optimal diabetic control normally with insulin
- Optimal lipid control
- Use of aspirin, β blockers, ACE inhibitors as indicated

The histogram showing rates of serious cardiovascular events according to blood pressure in patients with hypertension and Type 2 diabetes is adapted from Hansson L, et al. *Lancet* 1998;351:1755-62. The figure showing Kaplan Meier estimates of the composite outcome of myocardial infarction, stroke, or death from cardiovascular causes in the HOPE study is adapted from Yusuf S, et al. *New Engl J Med* 2000;342:145-53. The figure showing simvastatin: vascular event by follow up duration is adapted from the Heart Protection Study website *www.ctsu.ox.ac.uk/~hps*. The table showing some causes of secondary hyperlipaedemia is adapted from International Task Force for Prevention of Coronary Heart Disease. *Nutr Metab Cardiovasc Dis* 1992;2:113-56.

18 Pregnancy

Fifty years ago, more than one quarter of diabetic pregnancies ended in fetal death. Now, due to major developments in obstetrics, diabetes, and paediatrics, most are successful, although perinatal mortality at 2 to 5% is still higher than normal (<1%). Major congenital malformations, some of which could be prevented by good preconception diabetes control, are still excessive.

Good results in diabetic pregnancy can only be achieved in centres where appropriate expertise exists. Joint clinics where care is shared between diabetes physicians and specialist nurses working alongside obstetricians with their team of midwives should be the norm. Attendance at separate clinics is a second-rate option: it is inconvenient and often confusing for patients and leads to inconsistent care and advice.

Management

Pre-pregnancy counselling
Education of diabetic women of childbearing age is important: they should be advised that if they plan a pregnancy they should attend a pre-pregnancy counselling clinic (ideally linked to the antenatal clinic), start taking folic acid and aim for optimal diabetic control before conception in order to reduce the incidence of congenital malformations. The goal is a HbA_{1c} < 6·5% although this is sometimes difficult to achieve even after several months of intense effort, and pragmatic decisions are often needed.

Pregnant diabetic women should report to their doctor or clinic as early as possible in pregnancy and be referred without delay to a joint diabetic antenatal clinic. The midwife should encourage them to attend their local antenatal classes for social contacts.

Congenital malformations
Pregnancy in Type 1 diabetes is associated with an increased risk of congenital malformations. There is a clear relationship between poor diabetic control in the first trimester, and it is equally established that optimal control before conception reduces the rate of congenital malformations to near normal. Thus an HbA_{1c} more than 50% above the upper limit is associated with a two to fourfold increase in the abnormality rate. While in a non-diabetic population congenital malformations occur in 1 to 1·5% of pregnancies, this may be as high as 4 to 6% in those with diabetes, or even higher in those with exceptionally poor control during the first trimester.

The abnormalities are essentially the same as those occurring in the general population and include skeletal abnormalities such as spina bifida or hemivertebra, congenital heart disease, and neurological defects such as microcephaly or anencephaly. Sacral agenesis is greatly increased in diabetes but is still very rare.

Tight control of diabetes before and during pregnancy
Diabetic control should be optimal throughout pregnancy; if it is not, admission to hospital, even for short spells, should be arranged without delay. Home blood glucose monitoring is performed at least four times daily to determine preprandial readings, and about one and a half hours after the main meals perhaps twice weekly to determine postprandial levels,

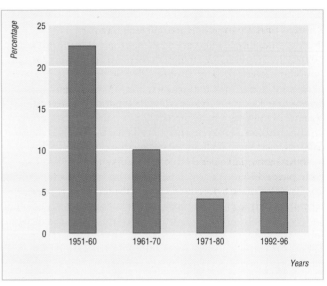

Diabetic pregnancies: perinatal mortality—King's College Hospital

Management of pregnancy and diabetes
- Pre-pregnancy counselling: understanding the need for tight diabetic control before conception, the need to take folic acid and of the commitment required for a good outcome
- Tight control of diabetes through pregnancy
- Management of diabetic complications during pregnancy
- Obstetric requirements and monitoring during pregnancy
- Management of diabetes in labour
- Management of the neonate

The incidence and relative risk of congenital malformations* in infants of diabetic mothers

Malformation	Incidence/1000 births	Relative risk compared with infants of non-diabetic mothers
Cardiac	10	4
Anencephaly	3	5
Arthrogryphosis	0.3	28
Ureteral duplication	0.7	23
Cystic kidney	0.6	4
Renal agenesis	0.3	5
Anorectal atresia	0.3	4
Caudal regression	1.3	212
Pesudohermaphroditism	0.6	11

*Thought to be of greater incidence in infants of diabetic mothers than in infants of non-diabetic mothers

especially when optimal HbA$_{1c}$ levels have not been achieved. Insulin injections are usually needed three or four times daily and patients should be taught how to adjust their own insulin doses. The dose of insulin needed often increases substantially during pregnancy, sometimes to twice or three times the usual amount and this needs to be anticipated. Good blood glucose control can be difficult to attain during the first trimester and attempts to do so are often complicated by severe hypoglycaemic episodes; thereafter most patients find that they can reach the standards of tight control without difficulty and without untoward hypoglycaemia. Suitable insulin regimens for tight control are described on page 21. Where serious difficulties (including severe hypoglycaemia) in achieving optimal control are encountered, continuous subcutaneous insulin infusion should be considered (see page 28-9). These patients and their families should be equipped with all the essential materials needed to cope with hypoglycaemia (see pages 34-5).

Type 2 diabetic pregnant women are increasingly seen especially among ethnic minorities. Treatment is by diet or diet and insulin only. Those who are on oral hypoglycaemic drugs should be changed to insulin, preferably before conception. There is however no evidence that tablet treatment is teratogenic, and where circumstances demand (for example, in countries where insulin is not readily available, or for patients who absolutely refuse insulin) they can be used. Indeed the use of glyburide has been examined and from a single large study in gestational diabetes appears safe, effective and, unlike some other sulphonylureas, does not cross the placenta, thus not provoking neonatal hypoglycaemia.

Management of diabetic complications during pregnancy

Retinopathy
Fundi should be examined routinely at the beginning, middle and end of pregnancy. If retinopathy is present early in pregnancy, more frequent examination is needed because occasionally progression is rapid during the course of pregnancy. If proliferative changes are present photocoagulation should be performed urgently.

Nephropathy
Patients with established proteinuria from nephropathy can expect problems during pregnancy, with an increased risk of fetal loss. When this is considered, together with the knowledge that the mother may need dialysis or transplantation within a few years, many of these patients should be advised to avoid pregnancy. However, with skilful management, most such patients whose renal function is still normal or near normal can expect a live infant. If however the serum creatinine exceeds 200 mmol/l the outlook for the fetus is bleak and patients should be strongly advised not to get pregnant.

Nephropathy and antihypertensive treatment
Patients with nephropathy who become pregnant can expect to become hypertensive and later often develop severe oedema. Fetal growth may be retarded, and because the problems can be severe, very early delivery of exceptionally small infants becomes necessary. With modern intensive neonatal care, most babies now survive, though a significant proportion develop mild or occasionally severe disabilities. Hypertension is treated with methyldopa, hydralazine, or occasionally labetalol or amlodipine. Frusemide can be given if a diuretic is needed, but

Preprandial blood glucose values should be maintained as near normal as possible and should preferably be kept below 4·0 to 5·5 mmol/l, though postprandial levels, which should be checked especially when HbA$_{1c}$ is suboptimal, may be up to 7·0 mmol/l. The target for HbA$_{1c}$ should ideally be within the normal range—that is, <6% if possible, although on occasions levels up to 7% represent the best that can be achieved

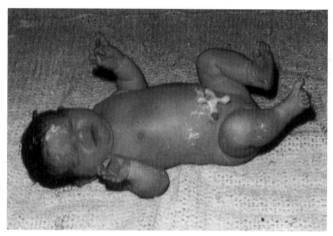
A typically large baby born to a diabetic mother

Diabetic women with established nephropathy should normally be advised against pregnancy. If the serum creatinine exceeds 200 µmol/l, the outlook for the fetus is very poor indeed

thiazides are contraindicated. Patients taking angiotensin converting enzyme inhibitors should be changed to other antihypertensive agents before pregnancy because of very serious later adverse effects on the fetus during pregnancy, though congenital malformations are not increased. Any patient with proteinuria from nephropathy may need protracted inpatient care, which should be undertaken in a specialist unit.

Obstetric requirements through pregnancy

An early ultrasound scan establishes the exact gestational age and detects major fetal abnormalities. A specific congenital abnormality ultrasound scan is required before 20 weeks. Thereafter a monthly scan documents the rate of fetal growth. There is considerable acceleration of growth after 28 weeks in the majority of diabetic pregnancies, even in the presence of good diabetic control. Retarded growth may be serious and requires specialist investigation. Assessment of fetal size and weight is important in determining the timing and mode of delivery.

Management in labour

Most patients should be admitted for a short period before planned delivery or for a longer period if there are either obstetric or diabetic problems. Fetal heart rate and its beat-to-beat variations are monitored regularly by an instantaneous heart rate meter and in cases of fetal distress other investigations are needed. Delivery is planned to take place as near to term as possible, unless there are medical or obstetric indications for earlier induction. The aim is for a vaginal delivery whenever possible. However, delivery is still on average at 37 weeks and about two-thirds of deliveries are still by caesarean section.

Glucose and insulin in labour
Glucose and insulin are given by intravenous infusion for all vaginal deliveries as follows:

Intravenous dextrose (10%): one litre every eight hours delivered at a steady rate.

Intravenous insulin: soluble insulin diluted in physiological saline (1 unit insulin/ml saline) and administered by infusion pump at about 1 unit/h (usual range 0·5-2 units/h). If very low infusion rates are used the insulin concentration can be halved.

Blood glucose concentrations should be maintained in the range 4·0-7·0 mmol/l. Insulin infusion is continued until the patient can restart her normal meals. The pre-pregnancy insulin dose is then restarted, otherwise severe hypoglycaemia will occur; if the patient was not previously on insulin, the insulin dose is halved.

Premature labour
Because of the hazards of premature labour, attempts may be made to promote fetal lung maturity by giving dexamethasone. This causes severe hyperglycaemia unless an intravenous insulin infusion is started at the same time as the administration of dexamethasone. Large doses of insulin may be needed.

Caesarean section
Insulin infusion is always used, as described in the section on management during surgery (see page 40).

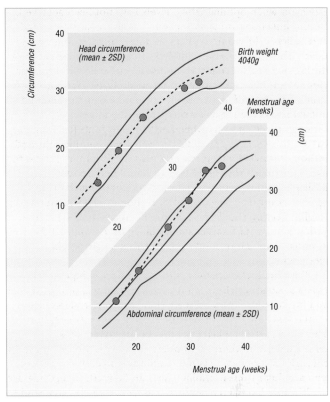

Ultrasound measurement of fetal growth showing excessive increase of abdominal girth, indicating delivery of a large baby

Blood glucose regimen in labour

Blood glucose	Infusion rate
<4·0 mmol/l*	0·5 U/h
4·0-7·0 mmol/l	1 U/h
>7·0 mmol/l	2 U/h

*If the blood glucose concentration decreases to <3·0 mmol/l, insulin infusion can be stopped for up to 30 minutes.

> If dexamethasone is used in premature labour, insulin must be infused at the same time to avoid severe hyperglycaemia

The neonate

The babies of diabetic mothers are larger than normal and nearly one-third of those with Type 1 diabetes exceed the 97·5% centile. However they no longer need care routinely in special care baby units unless there are specific reasons. Respiratory distress syndrome is now rarely seen in these infants unless they are very premature. Blood glucose concentrations should be checked regularly, especially in jittery babies, because hypoglycaemia is still commoner than in the infants of non-diabetic mothers. Polycythaemia, hyperbilirubinaemia, and hypocalcaemia are also commoner among these infants.

Breast feeding

This is encouraged in diabetic mothers as in non-diabetic mothers. The mother's diet should be increased by about 50 g of carbohydrate daily and ample fluids taken. The insulin dose is not usually affected when these measures are followed. Breast feeding mothers should not use oral hypoglycaemic agents.

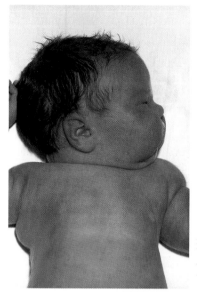

The neonate. "… they convey the distinct impression of having had such a surfeit of food and fluid pressed on them by an insistent hostess that they desire only peace so that they can recover from their excesses" (J. Farquhar)

Gestational diabetes (diabetes discovered during pregnancy)

The detection of gestational diabetes is undertaken by screening procedures in antenatal clinics. Babies born to women with gestational diabetes are frequently macrosomic and although both the effects on mortality and the benefits of intensive treatment are still uncertain, best practice requires optimal diabetic care for these patients.

Diagnosis

Routine blood glucose measurements are made in every pregnant woman between 26 and 28 weeks.

All women who have previously had gestational diabetes should have a glucose tolerance test between 26 and 30 weeks unless there are indications to perform it sooner.

Those from ethnic minorities carry a particularly high risk of gestational diabetes and at King's College Hospital those of African-Caribbean origin accounted for about 80% of them.

Treatment

Gestational diabetes is initially treated by diet alone. If control deteriorates using the criteria described above, insulin should be used, and stopped immediately on delivery of the infant. Oral hypoglycaemics are not advised, though there is no evidence that they are harmful.

Postpartum

A glucose tolerance test should be repeated six weeks after delivery. More than half of the patients return to normal; these women however have an approximately 50% risk of developing Type 2 diabetes later in life, sometimes within one year. An annual check of fasting blood glucose concentration is desirable, and they should be advised to avoid excessive weight gain by a regular programme of healthy eating and exercise (see chapter 3). Those patients who remain diabetic after pregnancy should be treated in the usual way.

Diagnosis of gestational diabetes

- A random plasma glucose concentration ≥11·1 mmol/l; fasting plasma glucose ≥7·0 mmol/l; whole blood glucose ≥6·1 mmol/l; are diagnostic of diabetes
- If a random blood glucose measurement is greater than 5·8 mmol/l perform a glucose tolerance test
- A 2 hour blood glucose ≥7·8 mmol/l during a glucose tolerance test in pregnancy is diagnostic of gestational diabetes

Contraception and diabetes

Good contraceptive advice for diabetic patients is vital to ensure that pregnancies are planned and conception takes place when diabetic control is optimal. All methods of contraception are available to diabetic women; the combined oral contraceptive pill is suitable in the absence of macrovascular disease or microvascular disease especially proteinuria, while progestogen-only methods provide a range of options including highly reliable long term methods, such as Depoprovera and implantable methods such as Implanon.

There is no evidence of any clinically significant effect on diabetic control from either combined oestrogen-progestogen pills or progestogen-only methods, nor is there any influence on the progression of diabetic complications. In the case of women with a history of gestational diabetes, the use of combined pills does not influence the subsequent development of Type 2 diabetes, but there is at present some doubt regarding the use of progestogen-only pills during lactation in women with recent gestational diabetes in whom there may be an increase in the subsequent incidence of Type 2 diabetes.

Intrauterine methods of contraception are suitable for women in stable relationships who have had at least one pregnancy, and may be ideal for diabetic women in whom hormonal (oestrogen containing) methods are contraindicated for either diabetic specific conditions or those unrelated to diabetes including cardiovascular or cerebrovascular disorders, venous thrombosis, pulmonary embolism or liver disease. Barrier methods of contraception have no metabolic consequences but are often insufficiently reliable, particularly if diabetic control is poor, when pregnancy should be rigorously avoided.

Sterilisation may be considered the ideal option when the family is complete, but it should be borne in mind that both Implanon and the progestogen delivering intrauterine system Mirena, provide more reliable contraception than laparoscopic sterilisation and are of course both reversible should circumstances change.

The table showing the incidence and relative risk of congenital malformations in infants of diabetic mothers is adapted from Combs CA, et al. *Clin Obstet Gynecol* 1991;5:315-31. The photograph of a typically large baby born to a diabetic mother is from Chamberlain G, Morgan M. *ABC of Antenatal Care*, 4th ed. London: BMJ Publishing Group, 2002.

The story of Mrs B-J continued: pregnancy

I had heard many tales about the trauma of diabetics who had babies, and I made up my mind I would never have any, even if I did get married. Once, when I was at the clinic, I was asked by the Sister if I would go up the maternity ward and have a chat with the two diabetic expectant mothers. They had been in hospital for nearly three months, which was normal in those days. The poor dears were bored stiff and glad to see a different face. I hope I cheered them up a bit. They convinced me that I would never want to follow their example and I never did. Dr Pyke told me a few years ago that things had changed now and expectant mothers no longer have to serve such a long sentence.

19 Organisation of diabetic care: primary-secondary care interface

Care of people with diabetes requires enthusiasm, commitment and organisation. There are various ways of undertaking it, but without interest and motivation, none will succeed.

It is best to bring diabetic patients together into properly organised clinics, whether in general practice or hospital, so that they can benefit from the wide range of services needed for their long-term care. A close liaison is needed between general practice and hospital specialists, and there are substantial new developments at the interface with Primary Care Groups and Primary Care Trusts. Patients can then have access to all members of the large team now involved in delivering the treatment and advice which they need. Diabetes shared care schemes are very advanced in many parts of the United Kingdom and set a model for other specialties, as they represent at the same time both efficient treatment and ideal links between hospitals and communities.

Any scheme aims to deliver the best care to patients. In order to do so there must be an efficient flow of information about patients, and the shared experience of a dedicated staff. Dissemination of expertise among all those concerned is essential. Schemes require nurturing, and an audit of outcome measures is needed for feedback to assess progress and identify courses of action. Local demographic trends must be understood, including an awareness of the needs of different ethnic groups. Education of the public is becoming increasingly important, and information is needed in schools as well. Research, innovation, and renewal are constantly needed. Increasingly, information regarding local diabetes services are provided on websites.

Requirements for diabetes care

A complex range of services for comprehensive diabetes care is needed as follows:

- to establish diagnosis and initiate treatment
- for patient education leading to independence
- to achieve optimal or appropriate diabetic control
- for screening and detection of diabetic complications
- to enable treatment of diabetic complications
- for care of those who are acutely or chronically ill
- for education of all medical and nursing staff involved in diabetes care.

The facilities needed to achieve these goals are provided by diabetes centres, which offer a common base for an integrated specialist and primary care diabetes service, and by the general practitioner.

Services provided by the general practitioner

- A diabetes register
- Dedicated time for care of people with diabetes
- Preferably one doctor with a special interest in diabetes
- A practice nurse who has received some specific training
- Access to all necessary laboratory services
- Facilities for complications screening and access to an eye screening programme
- Provision of access to the diabetes team to provide appropriate education, dietetic advice, and podiatry

---

St Vincent Declaration, 1989

A joint European initiative between the World Health Organization and the International Diabetes Federation resulted in the publication of the St Vincent Declaration in 1989, which calls for targets for improving the outlook for diabetic patients. The recommendations include:

- Reducing new blindness due to diabetes by a third or more
- Reducing numbers of people entering end stage diabetic renal failure by at least a third
- Reducing by a half the rate of limb amputations for diabetic gangrene
- Cutting morbidity and mortality from coronary heart disease in diabetic patients by vigorous programmes of risk reduction
- Achieving pregnancy outcome in diabetic women that approximates that of non-diabetic women

---

Services provided by diabetes centres

- Provide expertise, literature, and teaching aids based at the hospital department, and take the lead role in organisation of district diabetes services to co-ordinate hospital and general practitioner activities
- Provide mutually agreed guidelines on management
- Provide emergency access for patient and doctors (a direct, dedicated telephone line is essential)
- Establish a register of diabetic patients (and where possible also identify those at risk)
- The team should provide a clinical service for all new and established diabetic patients requiring specialist hospital attention
- Provide services jointly (ideally in joint clinics) with relevant specialists for the treatment of:
    Retinopathy with an ophthalmologist
    Pregnancy with obstetricians
    Children and adolescents with a paediatrician
    Foot problems (including peripheral vascular disease) with a vascular surgeon
    Renal problems with a nephrologist
    Neuropathy with a neurologist
    Erectile dysfunction
    Family and psychological problems
- Provide a screening service for detection of diabetic complications (see page 45)
- Oversee the care of all diabetic hospital inpatients by training ward-based "link" nurses
- Provide interpreters and patient advocates where necessary

The medical consultation

Every patient presenting for the first time should undergo a full clinical appraisal and physical examination. Subsequent consultations should not only include an assessment of the diabetes and its complications, but also specifically enquire regarding episodes of hypoglycaemia, supplementing this enquiry with reminders of how episodes should be managed and avoided. Inspection of insulin injection sites is often neglected. Assessment of other medical conditions and medication is also important because of potential interactions, and the need to offer each individual patient clinically appropriate advice.

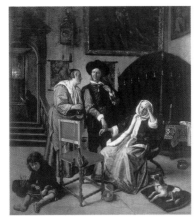

The Physician's Visit by Jan Steen, 1663

Indications for referral to the hospital diabetes centre

Good communications between community and hospital are crucial. While referral patterns will depend on local expertise, the following guidelines are offered:

Group 1 These patients should normally attend hospital diabetic clinics:

- Type 1 diabetic patients
- all children and adolescents with diabetes
- those with problems from hypoglycaemia
- patients who need pre-pregnancy counselling and all those who are pregnant
- patients with significant complications
- those with active foot lesions or sepsis, or both.

Group 2 Referral to hospital desirable, depending on local practice expertise:

- decision to commence insulin
- patients in whom adequate control is not achieved (for criteria see page 10)
- newly diagnosed patients for assessment, education, and initiation of treatment.

> **Urgent expert assistance (usually at the hospital diabetes centre is needed):**
> - If an active foot lesion develops
> - If there is a rapid decline of vision
> - For reappraisal after a serious hypoglycaemic event
> - If renal function deteriorates unexpectedly

The diabetes team

Because patient numbers are large, the disease lifelong, and its complications complex and diverse, a wide range of practitioners and specialists are involved in delivering a comprehensive service of high quality. The team needs a base, normally the diabetes centre in the local hospital, in order to maintain close communication with patients and professionals both in the hospital and in the community, as well as promoting innovation and research. Fragmented teams are likely to fail.

Diabetes specialist nurses and consultant nurses

The most important single innovation in diabetic care during the past three decades has been the increasing involvement of highly trained diabetes specialist nurses who can transform the standard of diabetic care, achieving liaison between hospital, general practitioner and patients at home, and offering a wide range of clinical and educational expertise. The Royal College of Nursing recommends that there should be one specialist nurse for a population of 50 000, and one for every 50 families with a diabetic child.

The training of nurses for diabetic care is of central importance and undertaken on specifically designed diploma and degree courses as well as at the diabetes centres themselves.

The diabetes team		
Diabetes centre	**General practice**	**Community**
Diabetes physician	General practitioner	
	Practice nurse	
Diabetes specialist nurse		
←	Dietitians →	→
←	Podiatrists →	→
←	Retinal screening staff →	→
Paediatrician		
Ophthalmologist		
Obstetrician		
Orthopaedic surgeon		
Vascular surgeon		
Renal physician		
Neurologist		
Psychologist		

The many important roles of the diabetes specialist nurse are closely linked to those of consultants, and can be summarised as follows:

- treatment of individual patients, linked with advice and counselling, establishing the right techniques and motivation needed to achieve proper diabetic management and control
- care of patients in hospital wards
- education of patients and professionals (see below)
- involvement in community care
- research, audit, and setting standards.

Consultant nurses have been established recently, with the aim both of enhancing clinical care and stimulating research and service innovations as well.

The role of the consultant in the community

The specialist diabetic consultant has a major role to play not only in the management of diabetes itself but also in the delivery of services across the community. Experience in the community surrounding King's College Hospital suggests the potential benefits of the following model seen in the box.

Education

Education of patients

An integral aspect of diabetes care is to inform all patients of the nature of the disorder and its treatment, and to place the potential threat of complications in their true perspective. Educational facilities are offered by the whole of the diabetes team both to individuals and to groups.

Instructions to new patients are always given initially on an individual basis. Most centres also organise courses for groups, ranging from a single half-day to comprehensive weekly series. There should be separate education groups for Type 1 and Type 2 diabetic patients, and the courses should provide scope for discussion and questions as well as direct instruction. Ongoing education is also needed to refresh memories over the several decades following diagnosis.

Education of patients has become very sophisticated in the field of diabetes; it has reduced admissions and to some extent complication rates, notably amputations. It is a concept which could be applied much more extensively to other areas of medicine.

Education of health professionals

In order to maintain standards, all those involved in diabetes care require regular updating, and every locality must take responsibility for educational programmes. These should include practice nurses, specialist nurses, hospital nurses, as well as junior and senior medical staff in both hospitals and general practice. Organisation of educational programmes requires a considerable resource.

Records

Computers are essential for the maintenance of good records on diabetes, though no single system is clearly superior. Maintenance of a register of diabetic patients is an essential operation and becomes increasingly important for recalling patients for review and assessment. Records of varying complexity can be held on the computer and the presentation can be structured so as to present the necessary information described below.

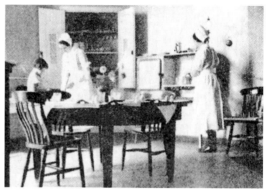

Diabetic kitchen, King's College Hospital, 1935 (Diabetes UK)

Role of the consultant

- The hospital team regularly visits general practices to see selected patients attending consultation
- The hospital team comprises a consultant and a diabetes specialist nurse, accompanied by a specialist registrar and a medical student
- The practice team includes the host general practitioners, practice nurses, and others such as local district nurses, health visitors, podiatrists, and dieticians

---

Aims of an education programme

- To explain the nature of the disease and its complications
- To explain the treatment, starting with the simplest ground rules and eventually provide comprehensive instructions on both treatment and monitoring, enabling patients to take control of their own condition
- To explain dietary and other lifestyle requirements
- To provide printed literature. "Starter" packs should contain:
  A booklet about diabetes
  Dietary instructions
  Home monitoring booklet with full instructions
  Information on driving
  Essential telephone numbers
  Leaflets on Diabetes UK

DIAMOND COMPUTER SYSTEM

Name

Hospital Number

D.O.B.:

Date	Weight	Body mass index	Systolic pressure	Diastolic pressure	Random blood glucose	HbA$_{1c}$	Creatinine	Albumin/ Creatinine ratio	Abustix	Cholesterol	Retinopathy		Visual acuity		Foot pulses		Feet
											R	L	R	L	R	L	
12/05/97	95.8	32.38	145	98	12.9	8.1	135	40.0	+ +		Laser	Laser	6/18	6/9	+	0	Healthy
10/02/97	97.7	33.02	130	80	13.9	10.7	72		+ +	6.8	Laser	Laser	6/18	6/9	+	0	Foot ulcer
16/09/96	100.5	33.97	150	94	11.8				+		Pre-prolif	Pre-prolif	6/6	6/6	+	+	
09/09/96	100.2	33.87	140	90	12.1	6.5	78		+ +		B'gd	B'gd	6/6	6/6			
11/03/96	97.1	32.82	130	85	4.6	6.3		3.4	Negative		B'gd	B'gd			+	+	Healthy
11/12/95	96.2		165	98	9.7	6.2	70	2.9	Trace	5.7	0	0	6/6	6/5			
01/12/93	90.6		110	78		11.2		0.2	Negative		0	0	6/6	6/5	+	+	Healthy

Patient history record

Special records are needed for proper care of diabetic patients both in hospital and in general practice—however this is organised, records must be immediately available when required. In hospital there are huge advantages in maintaining a separate set of records for diabetic patients and this system is used by major departments. Many general practices also keep special records supplementary to the basic "Lloyd George" card. Such records must be designed for serial recording of factual data, including weight, blood glucose, urine tests, HbA$_{1c}$, visual acuity, complications (results of eye examination in particular), and treatment. There must always be space for recording the outcome of the medical consultation itself and for treatment recommendations. There should be a system to alert the staff to the presence of particular problems, for example, sight-threatening retinopathy, and to the date when the next examination is required (for example, blood pressure measurement or eye examination). Many also incorporate an education checklist which records when patients have attended sessions and ensure that essential advice has been given, for example on driving.

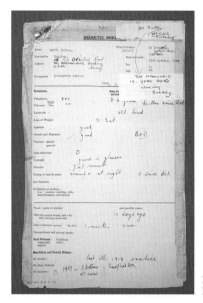

Early diabetic record in the hand of Dr R D Lawrence

Other facilities

Local diabetes service advisory groups (LDSAGs)

Coordination of services by LDSAGs is crucial to their success. Local committees can achieve this very effectively. They should comprise representatives of local purchasing authorities (for example health authorities or primary care trusts), providers (hospital consultants and general practitioners), diabetes specialist nurses, and consumers (diabetic patients). Effective discussions in this group can substantially enhance local services which might otherwise become seriously fragmented.

Diabetes facilitators

Support for general practices establishing diabetes services is crucial and a team for this purpose, comprising specialist nurses, facilitators, and a dietician, greatly enhances this process, assisting them with the development of optimal facilities and providing them with useful guidelines. The National Diabetes Facilitator's Group runs training courses.

Diabetes UK

The central resources of Diabetes UK provide direct advice for both patients and health professionals by printed literature, and access to scientific and epidemiological information. Diabetes UK also funds research, and provides scientific and educational meetings, children's camps, family weekends, and many other activities.

Local branches of Diabetes UK, organised by people with diabetes, serve as self help and fundraising groups, as well as helping to maintain high quality local services.

Juvenile Diabetes Research Foundation (JDRF)

This organisation was founded in the United States and is now established in the United Kingdom as well. Its chief aims are fund raising to support research, particularly in diabetes prevention and treatment, together with promotion of understanding of this condition by the public.

National Service Framework (NSF) for Diabetes: standards

The NSF for diabetes was published in 2002 and full details can be found on the website <www.doh.gov.uk/nsf/diabetes>

The standards have been divided into 12 sections relating to the following nine categories:

1 Prevention of Type 2 diabetes
2 Identification of people with Type 2 diabetes
3 Empowering people with diabetes
4 Clinical care of adults with diabetes
5 Clinical care of children and young people with diabetes
6 Management of diabetic emergencies
7 Care of people with diabetes during admission to hospital
8 Diabetes and pregnancy
9 Detection and management of long-term diabetic complications

---

Diabetes UK is at 10 Parkway, London NW1 7AA; telephone 020-7424-1000; <www.diabetes.org.uk>

The JDRF is at 19 Angel Gate, London EC1V 2PT; telephone 020-7713-2030 <www.jdrf.org.uk>

Conclusion

Obviously the requirements for diabetes care will vary from one geographical area to another, but anyone who undertakes the care of people with diabetes must heed the words of Dr Elliott P. Joslin: "To retain his patient for 20 years he must shun proprietary remedies as the devil does holy water, continually seek for new knowledge as eagerly as the diabetic grasps for life, but ever sift the wheat from the chaff remembering that faithful treatment in season and out of season is rewarded."

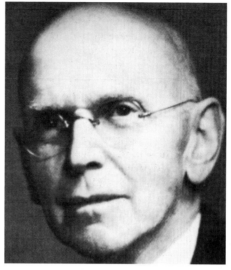

The Physician's Visit by Jan Steen, 1663 is reproduced with permission from the V&A Picture Library. The photograph of EP Josllin is from Joslin EP. *Diabetic Manual*, Lea and Febiger, 1941.

Elliott P Joslin, 1869-1962

The story of Mrs B-J continued: joining the Diabetic Association

I joined the Diabetic Association, as it was called then, when it was first formed (1934). Through them, I was sent to St Mary's Convalescent Home at Birchington to recuperate after the whooping cough attack. I was there for the Coronation of George VI in 1936, and can well remember the lovely party we had that day. My mother had sent me a parcel of patriotic items such as red, white and blue crepe paper, ribbons, and flowers made of red, white and blue feathers. With these I made myself an outfit for the fancy dress parade and won first prize, a china plate coronation souvenir.

The war brought problems for me and at the end of it, in 1945, I was quite run down. I think this was due to lack of fresh fruit, especially oranges and bananas. Diabetics were allowed to have three times the normal ration of meat, butter, margarine and cheese. To get this, the sugar ration had to be surrendered. Later in the war, when milk was rationed to two pints a week for each adult, diabetics were allowed one pint a day. Apart from the extra milk, I never had extra rations, as my mother witnessed an unpleasant scene one day in Sainsburys, and it put her off ever getting the extras; when a lady with three diabetics in her family was handed a large joint, there was almost a riot and the poor lady was manhandled and the meat torn away from her. The manager called the police to restore order. My mother was so upset that she firmly refused to apply to the Food Office for the permits and said that I would have her rations if necessary.

20 Practical problems

Employment and hobbies

Most of the problems of people with diabetes in society result from the ever present possibility of hypoglycaemia in insulin treated patients. Although this hazard is small in many individuals, it is an unacceptable risk in some circumstances. The guiding principles in making the difficult assessments for employment or hobbies relate to whether the risk of confusion during hypoglycaemia affects only the individual or whether it also places the safety of others at risk; the magnitude of the risk of diminished awareness of hypoglycaemia; and the magnitude of the hazard should a hypoglycaemia related accident occur.

Individual firms and industries have generally established their own regulations about the suitability of those with diabetes for particular jobs. If the candidates for employment are rejected unreasonably, solely on account of diabetes they may appeal. People with diabetes are not normally accepted by the armed forces, the police, or the merchant navy, and those already in these occupations may be diverted away from active service to office work. Shiftwork, especially nightshift work, should be avoided if possible by those taking insulin, but some patients can make appropriate adjustments and many may successfully cope with such work.

Diabetic people treated by diet alone or with oral hypoglycaemic tablets who are otherwise fit should be permitted to undertake any occupation or hobby. Their risk of hypoglycaemia is negligible.

Driving

All diabetic patients who are otherwise physically fit and not affected by blackouts, or other proscribed or relevant medical conditions, are normally allowed to hold ordinary Group 1 (category B) driving licences—that is, vehicles up to 3500 kg with up to nine seats and with a trailer up to 750 kg. The law demands that diabetic patients treated with tablets or insulin (but not those on diet alone) should inform the Driver and Vehicle Licensing Agency (DVLA) in Swansea. If applying for a licence for the first time, the appropriate declaration must be made on the application form. It is helpful to indicate whether insulin is being used. Driving licences are granted for three years and are reissued (at no extra fee) subject to a satisfactory medical report for those on insulin, and up to 70 years of age for those on diet or tablets, subject to any change of their health or treatment.

For any driving licence, visual acuity must be better than 6/12 in the better eye, and the visual field should exceed 120° horizontally and 20° above and below throughout 120°. Those who have had laser photocoagulation should report this to the DVLA so that appropriate visual field perimetry can be performed.

Healthy people with diabetes who are treated with diet or tablets are normally allowed to drive vehicles larger than those defined above (that is, Group 2), provided they pass a separate test to meet the higher Group 2 standards. Group 2 or vocational licences include those for large group vehicles and passenger carrying vehicles. Those taking insulin are not permitted to hold Group 2 licences, unless the license was granted before 1991 and subject to satisfactory medical reports, because of the serious potential consequences of hypoglycaemia, no matter how small the risk may be for any

Hypoglycaemia is the major hazard for any insulin treated diabetic patient

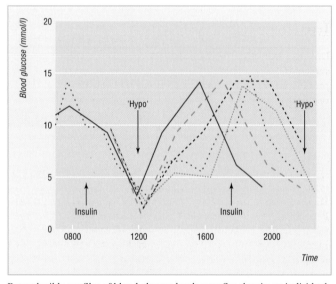

Reproducible profiles of blood glucose levels over five days in an individual patient, showing times when there is a risk of hypoglycaemia

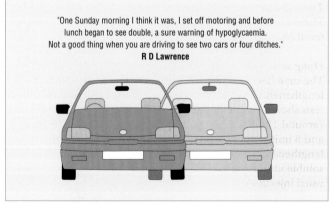

"One Sunday morning I think it was, I set off motoring and before lunch began to see double, a sure warning of hypoglycaemia. Not a good thing when you are driving to see two cars or four ditches."
R D Lawrence

Hazards when driving

individual diabetic patient. However, exceptional cases, based on individual assessment of the risk of experiencing diminished awareness of hypoglycaemia, can be identified (see Appendix 1) and enable some people to hold C1 licences (vehicles between 3500 and 7500 kg), although D1 vehicles (minibuses) do not fall into this category.

All insulin-treated diabetic patients who drive should always keep a supply of sugar in their cars. They should normally check blood glucose before driving, and should not drive if they are late for a meal, when the danger of hypoglycaemia is very great, especially around noon. If they experience warning symptoms of hypoglycaemia they should stop, switch off the ignition, and preferably leave the car, since they may otherwise be open to the charge of driving under the influence of drugs (insulin). Those unfortunate patients who are prone to hypoglycaemia without warning must not drive, and their doctors should make this advice very clear.

Insurance and pension

Driving insurance with a normal premium will usually be issued, subject to a satisfactory medical report. Life assurance premiums are often raised by amounts which depend on the result of a medical examination. It is worth looking for the "best buy". Sickness and holiday insurance premiums are often higher than normal. Diabetes UK offers helpful advice on insurance.

Travel

Diabetic control is easily upset by the rigours of travelling. People with diabetes should therefore undertake regular blood tests and adjust diet and insulin if necessary. Ideally those on insulin should travel with a companion if they are going to remote places. It is well worth carrying an identity disk which can be obtained from Diabetes UK, which also helps with appropriate foreign language leaflets. Some of the following circumstances present special problems.

Sea sickness and other stomach upsets causing vomiting
Diabetic patients may use the same anti-seasickness tablets as non-diabetics; these drugs do not change diabetic control. They do however tend to cause drowsiness, so it is best not to drive. If vomiting occurs insulin should be continued without fail and the situation dealt with as described on page 37.

Time changes on long-distance air travel
There are inevitably difficulties with diabetic control for a few days.

Flying west
The time between injections can, with little problem, be lengthened by two to three hours twice daily. Regular blood tests should be performed and if they are excessively high (around 15 mmol/l or more) extra soluble insulin (between 4 and 8 units) can be taken. If the time gap between injections is lengthened still further, a small supplementary injection of soluble insulin (between 4 and 8 units) is taken between the usual injections.

Flying east
The time between injections will need to be shortened by two to three hours each time, which could result in rather low blood glucose readings. Careful testing should be performed, and if required each dose can be reduced by a small amount

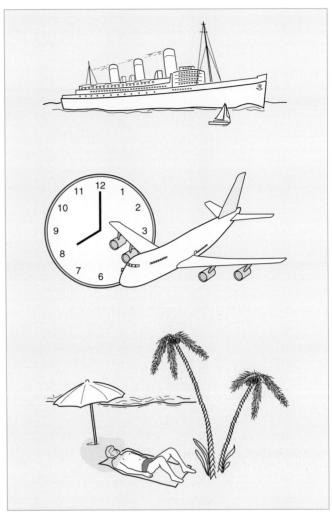

Hazards when travelling (sea sickness, time changes, burns on feet)

Other problems while abroad
- Vomiting either from motion sickness or stomach upsets (see page 37)
- Intercurrent illnesses affecting diabetic control, for example infections (see page 37)
- Hypoglycaemia (see page 34)
- Alterations of diabetic control due to major changes in diet or activity
- Burning feet on hot sand or stones, making foot protection with sandals or trainers extremely important

(4 to 8 units on average). Regular meals should be taken as normal. Many airlines will make special provision for those with diabetes if notified in advance; it is nevertheless strongly advisable to carry a food pack in case of delays or other emergencies.

Physical activity
More insulin may be needed if those with diabetes decide to be much less active when on holiday, or vice versa. Dietary indiscretions may also play havoc with control.

Breakage or loss of equipment
People with diabetes should carry ample supplies of syringes, insulin, needles, and testing equipment, and it is wise for a travelling companion to have a second set. The equipment in current use and that for emergency use is best kept in separate places. Soluble and isophane insulins are obtainable in most countries.

Storage of insulin
In a temperate climate insulin will keep for some months at room temperature (and furthermore injections sting less if the insulin is not chilled). Refrigeration is wise for prolonged visits to a tropical climate, and is also recommended for stocks kept at home for long periods, although exposed insulin actually deteriorates very little. Insulin should never be deep frozen and should not be left in the luggage hold of an aircraft, where it may freeze. Insulin is not damaged when passing through scanners.

Vaccination and inoculation
These are quite suitable for diabetic people and should be given for the same indications as for non-diabetics.

Dental treatment

Diabetic people may receive dental treatment in the normal way and without any special arrangements, except in the case of insulin treated patients needing a general anaesthetic, when a short admission to hospital is the wisest course. Dental infections and abscesses can of course upset diabetic control as is the case with any other source of infection.

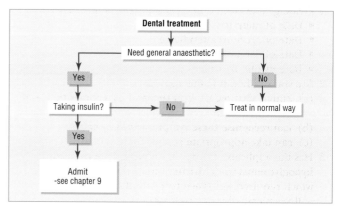

Dental treatment

The story of Mrs B-J concluded

I had started insulin only ten years after its discovery, but I remember meeting an elderly man in the upstairs waiting room by the path lab telling us that he had become diabetic before insulin, and how he thanked God for it every day. I know how he felt, but sadly his prophecy, that diabetes would be treated only like a cold in a further ten years, was not fulfilled.

During her early years Mrs B-J was treated with a variety of twice daily insulin regimens changing with the fashions of time and the whims of both herself and her physicians. The insulin dose in 1960 was around 26 units daily and in 2001 it is still approximately 24 units daily. Her HbA$_{1c}$ has ranged between 9% and 10% between 1995 and 2001-2.

At the time of writing early in 2002, Mrs B-J, now nearly 80 years old and with diabetes of nearly 70-years duration, still regularly attends the diabetic clinic at King's College Hospital and has done so without a break since 1932. Her medical records from 1932 are complete, and correspondence dates back to 1966.

Apart from the recent development of infection in one great toe, it is remarkable to observe that after all these years, she has no retinopathy (1999) and only mild lens opacities; there has never been any proteinuria and an absence of microalbuminuria was noted in 1999.

We must congratulate Mrs B-J for her courage and perseverance over so many years. We are grateful now for the privilege of being able to read the very personal account of her own diabetes which must give so much encouragement to others.

Appendix 1

Questionnaire to assess diminished awareness of hypoglycaemia

This questionnaire is recommended by the Driver and Vehicle Licensing Agency for applicants for certain driving licences as indicated on page 88 and is also of value in assessing patients involved in other hazardous activities or occupations. The applicant should be assessed by a consultant specialising in diabetes.

1 Please give details of medical supervision for diabetes.
   - Date of interview
   - Date of previous attendance
   - Date of diagnosis of diabetes
   - Date insulin treatment commenced
2 Are you satisfied that the applicant:
   (a) knows what symptoms can occur as a consequence of hypoglycaemia?
   (b) can recognise these symptoms if they occur?
   (c) can take appropriate action?
3 Has the applicant, to your knowledge, experienced hypoglycaemia while driving within the last 12 months, which required assistance from another person?
   If yes please give details/date(s):

4 Is there evidence of impaired awareness of hypoglycaemia in the past 12 months, during waking hours?
   If yes please give details/date(s):
5 Is there a history of hypoglycaemia during waking hours in the last 12 months requiring assistance from a third party?
   If yes please give details/date(s):
6 Does the applicant have a very clear understanding of diabetes and the necessary precautions for safe driving?
7 Does the applicant always carry an accessible supply of carbohydrate in the vehicle?
8 Does the applicant undertake blood glucose monitoring at least TWICE daily and at times relevant to driving on their current entitlement?
9 Have you examined the applicant's blood glucose records for the past three months?
   If no please explain why this was not done:
10 Are you satisfied with the accuracy of the results?
   If no, please explain why not:
11 Is there evidence of biochemical hypoglycaemia without symptoms (blood glucose below 3·0 mmol/l) on routine testing?
   If yes please give details:
12 Is there any diabetic complication or other medical condition that could affect safe driving?

Further information

Diabetes associations for patients and health professionals

American Diabetes Association (Patient and Professional),
1660 Duke Street,
Alexandria,
Virginia VA 22314,
USA.
Tel: 001-703-549-1500
Fax: 001-703-549-6995

Australian Diabetes Society (Professional),
145 Macquarie Street,
Sydney, NSW 2000,
Australia.
Tel: 0061-9256-5462
Fax: 0061-9251-8174
<www.racp.edu.au> e-mail <sneylon@racp.edu.au>

Diabetes UK (Patient and Professional),
10 Parkway,
London NW1 7AA,
UK.
Tel: 0044-20-7424-1000
<www.diabetes.org.uk>

Canadian Diabetes Association (Patient and Professional),
PO Box 12013,
Station BRM B,
Toronto, Ontario, M7Y 2L3,
Canada.
<www.diabetes.ca>

Diabetes Australia (Patient),
1st Floor Churchill House,
218 Northbourne Avenue,
Braddon ACT 2612,
Australia.
<www.diabetesaustralia.com.au>

Diabetes New Zealand (Patient),
PO Box 54, 1 Conquest Street,
Oamaru,
New Zealand.
<www.diabetes.org.nz> e-mail <info@diabetes.org.nz>

European Association for Study of Diabetes (Professional),
Rheindorfer Weg 3, D-40591,
Dusseldorf,
Germany.
Tel: 0049-211-7584690
Fax: 0049-211-75846929
<www.easd.org>
e-mail <easd@uni-dusseldorf.de>

Diabetes Federation of Ireland (Patient),
76 Lower Gardiner Street,
Dublin 1,
Ireland.
Tel and fax: 00353-1836-3022

Juvenile Diabetes Research Foundation International,
120 Wall Street,
New York,
NY 10005-4001,
USA.
Tel: 001-212-785-9595
<www.jdrf.org/index.php>

Juvenile Diabetes Research Foundation,
19, Angel Gate,
London, ECIV 2PT,
UK.
Tel: 0044-20-7713-2030
Fax: 0044-20-7713-2031
<www.jdrf.org.uk>

National Diabetes International Clearing House,
Box NDIC,
1 Information Way,
Bethesda,
MD 20892-3560,
USA.

New Zealand Society for the Study of Diabetes (Professional),
East Riding,
Whiterocks Road,
6-D RD Oamaru,
New Zealand.
Tel and fax: 0064-343-48110

Society for Endocrinology, Metabolism and Diabetes of South Africa (Professional),
PO Box 783155,
Sandton 2146,
Johannesburg,
South Africa.
Tel: 0027-11/202-0500
Fax: 0027-11/807-7989
e-mail <rsh@novonordisk.com>

South African Diabetes Association (Patient),
PO Box 3943,
Cape Town 8000,
South Africa.
<www.sada.org.za>

Useful websites

Clinical Standards for Diabetes (Scotland)	<www.clinicalstandards.org>
Exeter Genetic Screening Service	<www.diabetesgenes.org>
Heart Protection Study	<www.hpsinfo.org>
National Service Framework for Diabetes	<www.doh.gov.uk/nsf/diabetes>
Scottish Intercollegiate Guidelines Network (SIGN)	<www.sign.ac.uk>
Warwick Centre for Diabetes Education and Research	<www.diabetescare.warwick.ac.uk>

Further reading

Alberti KGMM, Defronzo RA, Keen H, Zimmet P, eds. *International Textbook of Diabetes Mellitus, 2nd ed.* Chichester: John Wiley & Sons Ltd, 1997. [A two volume comprehensive review.]

Amiel S. Is there anything new about insulin therapy? In: Amiel S, ed. *Horizons in Medicine.* Royal College of Physicians of London, 2002.

Angel A, Dhalla N, Pierce G, Singal P. *Diabetes and cardiovascular disease.* Netherlands: Kluwer Academic Publishers, 2001.

Besser GM, Bodansky HJ, Cudworth AG. *Clinical Diabetes: An Illustrated Text.* Philadelphia: JB. Lippincott, 1988. [An extensively illustrated text.]

Bilous R. HOPE and other recent trials of antihypertensive therapy in Type 2 diabetes. In: Amiel S, ed. *Horizons in Medicine.* Royal College of Physicians of London, 2002.

Bliss M. *The Discovery of Insulin.* Edinburgh: Paul Harris Publishing, 1983. [A masterful account of the events surrounding the discovery of insulin.]

Bloom A, Ireland J. (with revisions by Watkins PJ). *A Colour Atlas of Diabetes, 2nd ed.* London: Wolfe Publishing Ltd, 1992.

Boulton AJM, Connor H, Cavanagh PR, eds. *The Foot in Diabetes, 3rd ed.* Chichester: John Wiley & Sons Ltd, 2000.

Bowker JH, Pfeifer MA, eds. *Levin and O'Neals the diabetic foot.* St Louis: Mosby, 2001.

Day JL. *Living with diabetes, 2nd ed.* Chichester: John Wiley & Sons Ltd, 2001.

Dornhorst A, Hadden DR, eds. *Diabetes and pregnancy.* Chichester: John Wiley & Sons, 1996.

Dyck PJ, Thomas PK, eds. *Diabetic Neuropathy, 2nd ed.* Philadelphia: WB Saunders Co, 1999.

Edmonds ME, Foster AVM. *Managing the diabetic foot.* Oxford: Blackwell Science, 2000.

Ekoe JM, Zimmet P, Williams R. *Epidemiology of diabetes mellitus.* Chichester: John Wiley & Sons Ltd, 2001.

Fox C, Pickering A. *Diabetes in the real world.* London: Class Publishing, 1995. [A practical handbook advising on the needs of diabetic patients in general practice].

Frier BM, Fisher M, eds. *Hypoglycaemia.* London: Edward Arnold, 1993. [The most authoritative reference book on the subject at present.]

Frier BM, Fisher M, eds. *Hypoglycaemia in clinical diabetes.* Chichester: John Wiley & Sons Ltd, 1999.

Gill G, Pickup J, Williams G, eds. *Difficult diabetes.* Oxford: Blackwell Science, 2001.

Gill G, Mbanya J-C, Alberti G, eds. *Diabetes in Africa.* Cambridge: FSG Communications Ltd, Reach, 1997.

Hasslacher C. *Diabetic nephropathy.* Chichester: John Wiley & Sons Ltd, 2001.

Hollingsworth DR. *Pregnancy, Diabetes and Birth: a Management Guide, 2nd ed.* London: Williams and Wilkins Ltd, 1991.

Jeffcoate W, MacFarlane R. *The Diabetic Foot: An Illustrated Guide to Management.* London: Chapman and Hall, 1995.

Kahn CR, Weir GC, eds. *Joslin's Diabetes Mellitus.* Philadelphia: Lea and Febiger, 1995.

Kelmark CJH. *Childhood and Adolescent Diabetes.* London: Chapman and Hall, 1994.

Kirby R, Holmes S, Carson C. *Erectile dysfunction, 2nd ed.* Oxford: Health Press, 1999.

Krentz AJ, Bailey CJ. *Type 2 diabetes in practice.* London: Royal Society of Medicine Press Ltd, 2001.

Leslie RDG, Robbins DC, eds. *Diabetes: Clinical Science in Practice.* Cambridge: Cambridge University Press, 1995.

MacKinnon M. *Providing Diabetes Care General Practice, 4th ed.* London: Class Publishing, 2002.

Malins JM. *Clinical Diabetes Mellitus.* London: Eyre and Spottiswoode, 1968. [A splendid clinical description of diabetes.]

Mathias CJ, Bannister R, eds. *Autonomic Failure, 4th ed.* Oxford: University Press, Oxford, 1999.

Mogensen CE, ed. *The Kidney and Hypertension in Diabetes Mellitus, 5th ed.* USA: Kluwer Academic Publishing, 2000.

Nattrass M. *Malins' Clinical Diabetes, 2nd ed.* London: Chapman and Hall, 1994.

Page S, Hall G. *Diabetes: emergency and hospital management.* London: BMJ Publishing Group, 1999.

Pickup JC, Williams G, eds. *Textbook of Diabetes, 2nd ed.* Oxford: Blackwell Scientific Publications, 1997. [A substantial account in two volumes; beautifully illustrated.]

Pickup JC, Williams G. *Chronic Complications of Diabetes.* Oxford: Blackwell Scientific Publications, 1994. [A one volume updated version taken from the authors' two volume textbook.]

Ritz R, Rychlik I, eds. *Nephropathy in Type 2 diabetes.* Oxford: Oxford University Press, 1999.

Shaw KM, ed. *Diabetic complications.* Chichester: John Wiley and Sons, 1996.

Sinclair A, Finucane P. *Diabetes in old age, 2nd ed.* Chichester: John Wiley & Sons Ltd, 2000.

Tooke J, ed. *Diabetic angiopathy.* London: Arnold, 1999.

Warren S, Le Compte PM, Legg MA. *The Pathology of Diabetes Mellitus.* London: Henry Kimpton, 1966. [A classic account.]

Watkins PJ. The diabetic traveller. In: Dawood R, ed. *Travelers' Health.* Random House, New York, 2002.

Watkins PJ, Amiel S, Howell SL, Turner E. *Diabetes and its management, 6th ed.* Oxford: Blackwell Science, 2003.

West KM. *Epidemiology of Diabetes and its Vascular Lesions.* New York: Elsevier, 1978. [A classic review of diabetes in a world setting.]

Williams R, Wareham N, Kinmonth AM, Herman WH. *Evidence base for diabetes care.* Chichester: John Wiley & Sons Ltd, 2002.

Young A, Harries M, eds. *Physical activity for patients: an exercise prescription.* London: Royal College of Physicians, 2001.

United Kingdom Prospective Diabetes Survey (UKPDS). Original publications in *BMJ* and *Lancet*, September 1998.

Journal references

Atkinson MA, Eisenbarth GS. Type 1 diabetes: new perspectives on disease pathogenesis and treatment. *Lancet* 2001;358:221-9.

Barnett AH, Eff C, Leslie RDG, Pyke DA. Diabetes in identical twins: a study of 200 pairs. *Diabetologia* 1981;20:87-93.

Barrett T. Inherited diabetic disorders. CME Bulletin Endocrinology and Diabetes 1999;2:47-50.

DCCT: Diabetes Control and Complications Research Group. The effect of diabetes on the development and progression of long-term complications in insulin dependent diabetes. *New Engl J Med* 1993;329:977-86.

DIGAMI Study Group. Prospective randomised study of intensive insulin treatment on long-term survival after acute myocardial infarction in patients with diabetes mellitus. *BMJ* 1997;314:1512-15.

Euclid Study Group. Randomised placebo-controlled trial of lisinopril in normotensive patients with insulin dependent diabetes and normoalbuminuria or microalbuminuria. *Lancet* 1997;349:1787-92.

Expert Committee on the Diagnosis and Classification of Diabetes mellitus. Report of the Expert Committee on the Diagnosis and Classification of Diabetes. *Diabetes Care* 1997;20:1183-97.

Heller SR. Sudden cardiac death in young people with diabetes. *CME Bulletin Endocrinology and Diabetes,* 2000;3:4-7.

HOPE study: Heart Outcomes Prevention Evaluation Study Investigators. Effects of ramipril on cardiovascular and microvascular outcomes in people with diabetes mellitus. *Lancet* 2000;355:253-9.

Hoppener JWM, Ahren B, Lips CJM. Islet amyloid and Type 2 diabetes. *New Engl J Med* 2000;343:411-19.

MRC/BHF Heart protection study of cholesterol lowering with simvastatin in 20536 high-risk individuals: a randomised controlled trial. *Lancet* 2002;360:7-8

Owens DR, Zinman B, Bolli GB. Insulins today and beyond. *Lancet* 2001;358:739-46.

Ritz E, Orth SR. Nephropathy in patients with Type 2 diabetes. *New Engl J Med* 1999;341:1127-33.

Index

Page numbers in *italic* type refer to material in boxes or illustrations

Index

Index

Index

The complete ABC series

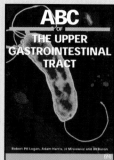

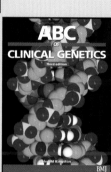

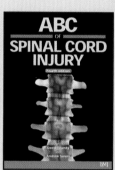

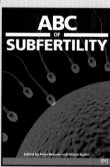

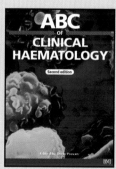